Sleep Apnea

The Essential Guide to Cure Your Sleep Apnea

(The Most Effective Tips and Tricks You Need to Know for Sleep Better)

Theo Gutierrez

Published By **Kate Sanders**

Theo Gutierrez

Sleep Apnea: The Essential Guide to Cure Your Sleep Apnea (The Most Effective Tips and Tricks You Need to Know for Sleep Better)

ISBN 978-1-7776902-0-5

No part of this guidebook shall be reproduced in any form without permission in writing from the publisher except in the case of brief quotations embodied in critical articles or reviews.

Legal & Disclaimer

Table Of Contents

Chapter 1: Understanding Sleep Apnea

Sleep apnea is a not unusual and probably intense sleep problem that influences tens of loads of hundreds of human beings global. It is essential to have a easy expertise of this situation to apprehend its signs and symptoms, are searching for appropriate analysis, and pursue powerful treatment.

Sleep apnea is characterised through using repeated pauses in respiration or shallow breaths at some point of sleep. These pauses, called apneas, can closing anywhere from a few seconds to severa mins and may take place over and over at some point of the route of the night time. There are three number one varieties of sleep apnea:

Obstructive Sleep Apnea (OSA): This is the most common form of sleep apnea. In spite of an try to respire, it takes place whilst the muscle corporations inside the returned of the throat are not able to preserve the airway open. The collapsed or blocked airway ends in reduced airflow or entire cessation of respiration.

Central Sleep Apnea (CSA): This shape of sleep apnea is an awful lot less commonplace and consists of a malfunction in the mind's respiration control center. It fails to ship the suitable signs and symptoms to the muscle organizations that control respiratory. Consequently, the individual may additionally revel in pauses in respiration.

CompSA, or complicated sleep apnea syndrome, is: Combining each obstructive and critical sleep apnea, CompSA is regularly known as remedy-emergent CSO.. It normally starts as obstructive sleep apnea but transitions into primary sleep apnea with continuous super airway pressure (CPAP) remedy.

The common symptoms and signs of sleep apnea encompass loud and persistent loud night breathing, immoderate daylight sleepiness, gasping or choking sooner or later of sleep, morning headaches, hassle concentrating, irritability, mood modifications, and burdened sleep. It is essential to be conscious that not truely absolutely everyone with sleep apnea will snore, and no longer all snorers have sleep apnea. Therefore, a whole evaluation thru way of a healthcare professional is crucial for an accurate evaluation.

Sleep apnea will have essential results on common fitness and well-being if left untreated. It has been associated with an prolonged hazard of high blood pressure, coronary coronary heart daylight accidents due sickness, stroke, diabetes, weight issues, and

If sleep apnea is suspected, a sleep have a observe, both performed at home or in a snooze lab, is generally encouraged for correct assessment. Treatment options for sleep apnea embody way of existence adjustments, on the side of weight reduction and positional remedy, as well as the usage of sleep apnea gadgets like continuous high-quality airway pressure (CPAP) machines, bi-degree excellent airway stress (BiPAP) machines, oral home equipment, and surgical interventions.

In cease, know-how sleep apnea is crucial for early reputation and

Recognizing the

powerful manipulate of

symptoms and signs and signs and symptoms, on the lookout for correct

the state of affairs. Diagnosis, and

pursuing appropriate treatment alternatives can considerably beautify sleep terrific, reduce associated health dangers, and beautify trendy well-being. If you believe you studied you or a person you recognize may also have

sleep apnea, it's miles endorsed to seek recommendation from a healthcare expert for assessment and steerage.

1.2 Types of Sleep Apnea

Sleep apnea is a snooze problem characterised through way of interruptions in

breathing for the duration of sleep. There are 3 number one kinds of sleep apnea: obstructive sleep apnea (OSA), good sized sleep apnea (CSA), and complex sleep apnea syndrome (CompSA).

The most commonplace sort of sleep apnea is known as obstructive sleep apnea, or OSA. It takes location at the same time as the muscle organizations in the decrease decrease lower back of the throat fail to keep the airway open, fundamental to repeated blockages or narrowing of the airway during sleep. These blockages, known as apneas, can bring about reduced airflow or entire cessation of respiratory. OSA is often associated with loud snoring, gasping, or choking all through sleep.

Central Sleep Apnea (CSA): CSA is much less common and takes place whilst the mind fails to ship the proper indicators to the muscle groups that manipulate respiratory. There isn't always any actual obstruction in the airway, in contrast to OSA. Instead, the respiration control center in the brain fails to initiate or regulate the breathing method. CSA is regularly associated with a loss of respiration strive and might cause disruptions in sleep styles.

Complex Sleep Apnea Syndrome (CompSA): CompSA, additionally called treatment-emergent applicable sleep apnea, is a combination of both OSA and CSA. It commonly starts offevolved as OSA but transitions into CSA with the use of non-stop exquisite airway pressure (CPAP) treatment. CompSA can pose unique disturbing situations in terms of remedy techniques and management.

It is critical to be aware that an entire assessment via a healthcare professional is essential to decide the appropriate form of sleep apnea a person can also moreover additionally have. The sort of sleep apnea identified could have an impact on the endorsed remedy alternatives, that can encompass way of life adjustments, using sleep apnea gadgets, or surgical interventions.

1.Three Symptoms and Health Risks

Sleep apnea is a sleep trouble characterized with the useful useful resource of interruptions in

respiratory for the duration of sleep. It is critical to understand the signs and apprehend the related fitness dangers to are seeking out appropriate analysis and treatment. Here are the common symptoms and fitness risks of sleep apnea:

Symptoms:

Loud and Chronic Snoring: Snoring is a favored symptom of sleep apnea, specifically in obstructive sleep apnea (OSA) times. The snoring is regularly loud, disruptive, and may be followed through pauses or gasping sounds.

Excessive Daytime Sleepiness: Individuals with sleep apnea often enjoy immoderate daylight hours sleepiness, feeling continuously worn-out, fatigued, or lacking electricity inside the direction of the day. This can cause troubles in hobby, memory problems, and impaired cognitive feature.

Gasping or Choking Sensations: People with sleep apnea may also additionally moreover awaken abruptly in the course of the night time with a sensation of gasping for air or choking. These awakenings are often fleeting and may not be detected. Morning Headaches: Sleep apnea sufferers might also additionally frequently awaken with headaches in the morning because of the intermittent interruptions in respiratory and the consequent lower in oxygen degrees during sleep.

Restless Sleep and Insomnia: Sleep apnea can cause disrupted and confused sleep patterns. Individuals can also discover themselves tossing and turning, waking up regularly throughout the night time time, and having hassle falling again to sleep.

Health Risks:

Hypertension (High Blood Pressure): Sleep apnea is associated with an stepped forward threat of excessive blood pressure. The repeated interruptions in respiratory purpose fluctuations in blood oxygen tiers, foremost to expanded blood pressure ranges.

Cardiovascular Disease: Sleep apnea is a chance aspect for diverse cardiovascular conditions, which encompass coronary coronary coronary heart disorder, coronary coronary heart assault, stroke, and atypical heart rhythms (arrhythmias).

The combination of oxygen deprivation, progressed blood strain, and the pressure on the cardiovascular system can make contributions to those dangers.

Type 2 Diabetes: Research has indicated a connection among sleep apnea and a higher hazard of kind 2 diabetes. The disrupted sleep styles and the impact on insulin resistance can also contribute to the development or worsening of diabetes.

Obesity: Obesity and sleep apnea regularly coexist, and there may be a bidirectional courting many of the 2. Obesity can growth the risk of developing sleep apnea, even as sleep apnea can contribute to weight gain and problem in dropping weight.

Daytime Fatigue and Impaired Quality of Life: The continual sleep deprivation and fragmented sleep attributable to sleep apnea can significantly impact an man or woman's remarkable of existence. Daytime fatigue, temper disturbances, irritability, and decreased productiveness are common effects.

Recognizing the signs and symptoms and knowledge the functionality fitness dangers associated with sleep apnea is essential for looking for clinical evaluation and pursuing control of sleep apnea suitable remedy. Effective can extensively beautify sleep top notch, lessen health risks, and enhance trendy properly-being. If you observed you or someone you understand may additionally additionally have sleep apnea, it's far advocated to speak over with a healthcare expert for evaluation and guidance.

1.Four Importance of Treatment

Sleep apnea is a excessive sleep trouble that requires well timed

prognosis and appropriate treatment. The significance of seeking out remedy for sleep apnea can not be overstated because of the potential health implications and the huge effect it may have on an character's everyday nicely-being. Here are key motives why treatment is critical for sleep apnea:

Improvement in Sleep Quality: Treatment for sleep apnea interests to repair regular respiratory patterns for the duration of sleep, which ends up in superior sleep first-rate. By addressing the underlying motives of sleep apnea and making sure uninterrupted breathing, people can enjoy restful and clean sleep, waking up feeling more energized and revitalized.

Reduction of Health Risks: Sleep apnea has been associated with severa health dangers, which include immoderate blood stress (immoderate blood stress), cardiovascular sickness, stroke, kind

weight problems. Effective treatment can help mitigate

2 diabetes, and

the ones risks via improving oxygenation, lowering blood pressure, and promoting cardiovascular fitness. It also can contribute to better glycemic control in people with diabetes.

Chapter 2: Continuous Positive Airway Pressure

2.1 What is CPAP?

CPAP, which stands for Continuous Positive Airway Pressure, is a common treatment technique for obstructive sleep apnea (OSA) and

specific respiratory-related sleep issues. CPAP treatment includes using a CPAP device that promises a non-prevent movement of pressurized air to keep the airway open sooner or later of sleep.

The CPAP machine includes three fundamental components: a motor, a humidifier, and a masks. The motor generates the pressurized air, it's miles introduced to the man or woman through a flexible tube. The air is humidified through the humidifier to save you dryness and infection of the airlines. The masks, which can be a nasal mask, nasal pillows, or a full-face masks, is worn over the nose and/or mouth to deliver the pressurized air right away into the airway.

The pressurized air from the CPAP device acts as a splint, effectively preserving the airway open and stopping collapse or obstruction in some unspecified time in the future of sleep. By maintaining a non-prevent and unobstructed airflow, CPAP remedy gets rid of or extensively reduces the apneas (pauses in breathing) and hypopneas (shallow respiratory) function of sleep apnea. This lets in individuals with sleep apnea to have uninterrupted and restful sleep, major to advanced sleep exquisite and daylight hours functioning.

CPAP remedy is generally prescribed based totally at the severity of sleep apnea and individual dreams. The prescribed stress level is decided all through a sleep have a have a look at or thru a CPAP titration have a study, which includes regularly growing the air pressure till the appropriate healing diploma is completed.

Benefits of CPAP remedy encompass:

Reduction in snoring: CPAP remedy lets in do away with or lessen snoring, offering consolation to bed companions and enhancing sleep exceptional for each human beings.

Improved sleep excellent: By preventing apneas and making sure non-forestall breathing, CPAP treatment promotes restful and undisturbed sleep, essential to extra suitable regular sleep satisfactory.

Alleviation of sunlight hours signs and symptoms and signs and symptoms: CPAP therapy can alleviate daylight sleepiness, fatigue, and cognitive impairments due to sleep apnea, resulting in extended electricity ranges and progressed daylight functioning.

Reduction of health risks: By efficiently treating sleep apnea, CPAP therapy permits lessen the related fitness dangers, together with immoderate blood stress, cardiovascular disease, stroke, and diabetes.

Enhanced great of life: With improved sleep, increased energy, and better ordinary health, CPAP remedy can positively impact an character's super of life, mood, and nicely-being.

It is crucial to artwork intently with a healthcare professional to determine the ideal strain settings, mask in shape, and ensure compliance with CPAP remedy. Regular examine-up visits and mask changes can be important to optimize comfort and effectiveness.

2.2 How CPAP Devices Work

CPAP (Continuous Positive Airway Pressure) gadgets are broadly used inside the remedy of obstructive sleep apnea (OSA) and one-of-a-type respiration-associated sleep troubles. These devices paintings with the resource of handing over a non-prevent bypass of pressurized air to the airway, successfully maintaining it open during sleep and stopping airway crumble.

The number one functioning of a CPAP device consists of three most important components: a motor, a humidifier, and a mask.

Motor: The motor is the middle thing of the CPAP tool. It generates a normal drift of pressurized air. The air is filtered to cast off impurities earlier than being pressurized through the motor.

Humidifier: Many CPAP gadgets encompass a humidifier problem. The humidifier provides moisture to the pressurized air, stopping dryness and irritation of the airlines. This permits to beautify comfort and reduce potential aspect outcomes, which encompass nasal congestion or dry throat.

Mask: The mask is worn over the nose, mouth, or every, and serves due to the fact the interface for turning in the pressurized air. There are one-of-a-type varieties of masks available, which incorporates nasal masks, nasal pillows, and complete-face mask. The masks is hooked up to the CPAP tool thru a flexible tube that gives the pressurized air from the motor to the masks.

When the CPAP device is grew to grow to be on and the mask is well ready, the pressurized air flows constantly into the airway. The progressed air pressure acts as a pneumatic splint, stopping the airway from collapsing in the direction of sleep. By preserving the airway open, CPAP remedy eliminates or drastically reduces the apneas (pauses in breathing) and hypopneas (shallow respiratory) associated with sleep apnea.

It is critical to determine the right pressure stage for each individual. This is generally carried out thru a snooze observe or a CPAP titration have a look at, which incorporates often developing the air pressure until the maximum fine recovery degree is achieved. The prescribed pressure setting guarantees that the air stress is sufficient to preserve an open airway and prevent breathing disruptions.

CPAP devices additionally feature numerous settings and functions to decorate person consolation and convenience. These can also encompass ramp talents that grade by grade increase the stress to the prescribed level, expiratory strain relief (EPR) to facilitate a lot much less tough exhalation, and facts recording capabilities for remedy effectiveness.

tracking compliance and

Overall, CPAP gadgets offer a non-invasive and effective

treatment method for sleep apnea. By turning in non-prevent excessive fantastic airway strain, those gadgets help human beings with sleep apnea attain restful sleep, alleviate symptoms and signs and symptoms and signs, and reduce the associated health dangers.

2.Three Types of CPAP Devices

CPAP (Continuous Positive Airway Pressure) therapy is a widely used treatment for obstructive sleep apnea (OSA) and one of a type breathing-related sleep problems.

There are remarkable kinds of CPAP gadgets to be had, every with its non-public competencies and variations. Here are the precept varieties of CPAP gadgets:

Standard CPAP: Standard CPAP devices supply a set degree of continuous air stress during the night time time. The prescribed strain is determined based totally surely on the severity of sleep apnea and man or woman goals. These devices are frequently the preliminary choice for treating sleep apnea and are appropriate for folks that require a constant strain putting.

Auto-Adjusting CPAP (APAP): Auto-Adjusting CPAP gadgets, additionally called AutoCPAP or APAP, constantly display and routinely modify the brought air pressure based totally at the person's breathing styles. These gadgets can dynamically modify the stress level in reaction to adjustments in the airway resistance at some point of sleep. APAP devices offer custom designed remedy thru providing the minimum powerful strain had to hold an open airway, making them appropriate for individuals with numerous pressure necessities.

Bi-Level Positive Airway Pressure (BiPAP): Bi-Level Positive Airway Pressure devices, furthermore known as BiPAP or BPAP, deliver precise stress tiers: a higher inspiratory strain sooner or later of inhalation and a lower expiratory pressure at some stage in exhalation. This dual stress feature presents greater comfort for people who find out it hard to exhale in the direction of the steady pressure of a famous CPAP device. BiPAP gadgets are regularly used for individuals with better stress necessities or precise respiratory conditions.

Travel CPAP: Travel CPAP gadgets are compact and transportable variations of preferred CPAP machines. These gadgets are designed for ease of journey and comfort, making them appropriate for individuals who want to apply CPAP treatment on the equal time as at the cross. Travel CPAP machines are normally smaller, mild-weight, and provide talents like battery operation and compatibility with notable power property.

It is essential to be conscious that a few CPAP devices might also consist of greater skills together with blanketed humidifiers, facts recording talents, mask leak detection, and advanced algorithms for detecting and responding to respiratory activities. These functions can enhance comfort, compliance, and remedy effectiveness.

The desire of CPAP tool is based upon on elements which encompass the severity of sleep apnea, character options, consolation, and precise remedy necessities. It is typically endorsed to go to a healthcare professional or a snooze expert to determine the maximum suitable CPAP tool and settings for powerful and cushty treatment.

2.4 Benefits and Limitations

CPAP (Continuous Positive Airway Pressure) devices are a appreciably used remedy preference for sleep apnea and different respiratory-associated sleep issues. These devices provide several benefits in dealing with sleep apnea symptoms and symptoms and improving ordinary nicely-being. It's crucial to apprehend their boundaries, despite the fact that. Here are the advantages and limitations of CPAP gadgets:

Benefits of CPAP Devices:

Effective Treatment: CPAP gadgets are quite powerful in treating sleep apnea via way of imparting a non-stop movement of pressurized air to maintain the airway open. This permits to eliminate or considerably reduce apneas and hypopneas, allowing human beings to breathe generally in the course of sleep.

Improved Sleep Quality: By maintaining an open airway, CPAP remedy promotes uninterrupted and restful sleep. This outcomes in advanced sleep superb, higher sleep architecture, and extra perfect daylight hours alertness.

Reduction in Symptoms: CPAP remedy can alleviate not unusual sleep apnea signs and symptoms and signs consisting of loud loud night breathing, sunlight hours sleepiness, morning headaches, and cognitive impairments. Additionally, it can enhance mood, reputation, and favored cognitive performance. Health Benefits: Treating sleep apnea with CPAP devices can have excellent influences on universal fitness. It can assist lessen the hazard of immoderate blood strain, cardiovascular sickness, stroke, and specific related fitness situations associated with untreated sleep apnea.

Customizable Treatment: CPAP gadgets can be adjusted and custom designed to satisfy person wishes. The pressure settings can be great-tuned primarily based on sleep have a take a look at outcomes and character comfort, making sure gold good sized treatment efficacy.

Limitations of CPAP Devices:

Mask Discomfort: Some humans can also enjoy pain or problem adjusting to carrying a CPAP masks. It might also additionally take time to discover the proper masks type and length that gives a snug healthy.

Mask Leak and Skin Irritation: Improper mask in form or insufficient protection can result in masks leak and pores and pores and skin contamination. Ensuring a right masks seal and working towards particular hygiene can help mitigate the ones problems.

Compliance Challenges: Consistent and lengthy-term use of CPAP devices might also moreover gift annoying conditions for some people. Factors which include mask pain, noise, claustrophobia, or issue adjusting to the treatment everyday can impact compliance.

Travel and Portability: Traditional CPAP devices won't be as transportable or reachable for tour. However, journey-specific

CPAP machines are available to deal with the ones boundaries.

Side Effects: Some people can also enjoy component results which embody dry mouth, nasal congestion, or bloating at the identical time as the usage of CPAP gadgets. Proper humidification and changes to pressure settings can assist control the ones thing outcomes.

It's vital to deal with any issues or problems with a healthcare expert or a snooze specialist to discover solutions and ensure powerful treatment. CPAP remedy can notably beautify sleep nice and trendy fitness at the same time as used continuously and in accordance with the advocated hints.

2.Five Tips for Using CPAP Devices

Using a CPAP (Continuous Positive Airway Pressure) device for sleep apnea treatment can extensively enhance sleep great and normal well-being. To maximize the effectiveness and luxury of CPAP treatment, right here are some useful recommendations for using CPAP devices: Proper Mask Fit: Ensure that your CPAP mask suits nicely and offers a cushty seal. A proper mask wholesome is crucial for effective remedy and to decrease air leaks. Work together with your healthcare company to select the proper mask type and length that suits your goals and opportunities.

Consistent Usage: Use your CPAP tool each time you sleep, together with naps. Consistent utilization is important for experiencing the complete benefits of CPAP therapy. Establish a ordinary and make CPAP utilization a regular a part of your sleep ordinary.

Humidification: If your CPAP tool has a integrated humidifier, use it to function moisture to the pressurized air. This can assist save you dryness or ache within the nasal passages and throat. Adjust the humidity diploma as favored for gold huge comfort.

Cleanliness and Maintenance: Follow the producer's commands for cleaning and retaining your CPAP machine. Regularly easy the masks, tubing, and humidifier to save you bacterial increase and ensure top-rated regular usual overall performance. Replace filters and different factors as encouraged.

Positioning: Sleeping in a snug position that allows you to preserve a exquisite masks seal is essential. Avoid slumbering on your belly or collectively along side your head at a clumsy perspective which can disrupt the masks seal or cause pain.

Noise Reduction: CPAP gadgets can produce some noise in the course of operation. If the noise is bothersome, recollect using a CPAP gadget with a noise cut price feature or putting the device in addition a ways from the bed.

Chapter 3: Level Positive Airway Pressure

3.1 What is BiPAP?

BiPAP, which stands for Bi-Level Positive Airway Pressure, is a type of respiration remedy used to address sleep apnea and exclusive respiratory-related issues. BiPAP devices deliver two special tiers of air strain: a better pressure inside the direction of inhalation (inspiratory terrific airway pressure or IPAP) and a decrease strain during exhalation (expiratory superb airway pressure or EPAP).

BiPAP remedy is frequently advocated for human beings who have difficulty exhaling inside the course of the regular strain introduced through a big CPAP (Continuous Positive Airway Pressure) device. The functionality to deliver particular pressure degrees at some degree within the breathing cycle makes BiPAP devices more tolerate for some people.

cushty and much less complex to

BiPAP treatment works thru the use of the use of a machine that has comparable

additives to a CPAP device, inclusive of a motor, a humidifier, and a mask. The motor generates the pressurized air, that is delivered to the consumer thru a tube linked to a masks worn over the nostril, mouth, or every.

During inhalation, the BiPAP device substances a higher stress (IPAP) to useful resource the airway and assist with respiratory. This higher strain allows conquer resistance or blockages in the airway. During exhalation, the stress is decreased (EPAP) to lessen the strive required to exhale. This pressure remedy sooner or later of exhalation can make breathing closer to the tool more snug and herbal.

The functionality to regulate the IPAP and EPAP settings makes BiPAP remedy customizable to everybody's wishes. This permits healthcare carriers to fantastic-track the remedy to offer ideal remedy efficacy.

BiPAP therapy is mainly useful for people with first rate breathing conditions, which incorporates weight problems hypoventilation syndrome, persistent obstructive pulmonary disorder (COPD), or complicated sleep apnea syndrome (CompSA). These situations frequently require better strain useful resource in the course of inhalation and might experience the stress comfort in some unspecified time in the destiny of exhalation.

It is essential to be conscious that BiPAP therapy requires a prescription from a healthcare corporation. A sleep test or a titration take a look at can be performed to decide the best strain settings for each individual.

Overall, BiPAP therapy gives an possibility treatment preference for people who also can have trouble tolerating CPAP treatment. By offering certainly one of a kind pressure ranges, BiPAP devices assist maintain open airlines, beautify breathing, and decorate conventional sleep great.

3.2 How BiPAP Devices Work

BiPAP (Bi-Level Positive Airway Pressure) devices are breathing

treatment devices usually used within the remedy of sleep apnea, respiratory insufficiency, and exclusive breathing-associated troubles. BiPAP devices paintings with the aid of way of delivering outstanding tiers of air stress: inspiratory powerful airway stress (IPAP) and expiratory effective airway stress (EPAP).

Here's how BiPAP devices paintings:

IPAP (Inspiratory Positive Airway Pressure): During inhalation, the BiPAP gadget offers a better strain referred to as IPAP. IPAP assists in beginning and supporting the airway, supporting humans with respiratory issues overcome resistance or blockages. This improved pressure promotes better air go together with the go with the flow and ensures an accurate sufficient deliver of oxygen.

EPAP (Expiratory Positive Airway Pressure): When the person exhales, the BiPAP tool reduces the pressure to a lower stage referred to as EPAP. This strain treatment inside the route of exhalation lets in for a whole lot much less complex and extra comfortable respiration.

By lowering the pressure, BiPAP gadgets assist in decreasing the effort required to exhale in competition to the non-prevent pressure generally professional with CPAP (Continuous Positive Airway Pressure) devices.

Dual Pressure Settings: The capability to alter IPAP and EPAP settings makes BiPAP treatment pretty customizable. Healthcare companies decide the precise strain person needs, regularly determined thru a degrees primarily based mostly on

sleep have a look at or titration check. The IPAP and EPAP settings may be tailor-made to cope with the severity of sleep apnea, breathing situations, or precise affected man or woman necessities.

BiPAP Machine Components: BiPAP gadgets embody a motor, a humidifier, a tubing gadget, and a masks. The motor generates pressurized air, that is brought to the client thru a tube related to the masks. The humidifier offers moisture to the delivered air, reducing potential dryness or inflammation inside the airlines.

Monitoring and Adjustments: BiPAP gadgets might also furthermore function monitoring abilities that song the man or woman's respiratory patterns and remedy adherence. This records can help healthcare groups test remedy efficacy and make important modifications to the stress settings through the years.

BiPAP treatment is commonly used for those who conflict with exhaling in the route of the ordinary strain of CPAP gadgets or require greater stress assist all through inhalation due to underlying respiration situations. The customizable stress settings of BiPAP devices enhance consolation and compliance, leading to advanced sleep pleasant, decreased signs and symptoms, and superior normal properly-being.

It is essential to visit a healthcare company or a nap expert to decide the most appropriate treatment and strain settings for an man or woman's particular dreams. Regular have a look at-up appointments and communique with the healthcare company are crucial to show remedy effectiveness and make any crucial changes.

three.Three Differences Between CPAP and BiPAP

CPAP (Continuous Positive Airway Pressure) and BiPAP (BiLevel Positive Airway Pressure) are every commonly used remedies for sleep apnea and wonderful respiratory-associated problems. While they've similar functions, there are tremendous variations among CPAP and BiPAP gadgets in phrases in their capability and applications:

Pressure Delivery: The key difference among CPAP and BiPAP lies in how they deliver air stress. CPAP devices offer a non-stop, constant stress at some degree within the respiratory cycle. On the opportunity hand, BiPAP gadgets supply two awesome degrees of stress: a higher inspiratory excessive first-rate airway stress (IPAP) all through inhalation and a decrease expiratory excellent airway strain (EPAP) at some point of exhalation. This twin stress feature of BiPAP allows for plenty much less difficult exhalation in competition to reduced stress, making it useful for people who have problem exhaling in opposition to the normal pressure of CPAP.

Treatment Applications: CPAP remedy is commonly prescribed for people with obstructive sleep apnea (OSA), in which the airway collapses or becomes blocked at some point of sleep. It helps to hold a consistent open airway through offering non-stop incredible stress. BiPAP remedy is frequently advocated for people with more complicated respiration situations, which include number one sleep apnea (CSA), respiratory insufficiency, or situations that require more help in the end of inhalation and reduced pressure for the duration of exhalation.

Treatment Tolerance: Due to the dual strain settings, BiPAP remedy is commonly considered more comfortable and less difficult to tolerate than CPAP, in particular for individuals who conflict with exhaling in opposition to regular pressure. BiPAP gives a smoother transition among inhalation and exhalation, making it more suitable for those with notable respiration conditions or sensitivities.

Prescription and Titration: Both CPAP and BiPAP treatments require a prescription from a healthcare agency. However, the way of identifying the right stress settings may furthermore variety. CPAP titration studies typically determine a fixed stress degree, at the same time as BiPAP titration studies recognition on establishing each IPAP and EPAP ranges primarily based on character needs.

Cost and Availability: In great, CPAP gadgets are greater broadly to be had and have a tendency to be more low-rate as compared to BiPAP gadgets. However, the deliver and charge of each CPAP and BiPAP gadgets can range relying on location, coverage insurance, and particular talents.

It's essential to be aware that the selection among CPAP and BiPAP is primarily based upon on character desires, sleep have a have a look at consequences, and the recommendation of a healthcare provider or sleep professional. The suitable treatment opportunity can be determined based on elements which incorporates the severity of the sleep trouble, underlying breathing conditions, and patient comfort. To verify the great course of remedy, talking with a healthcare expert is critical.

3.Four Suitable Candidates for BiPAP

BiPAP (Bi-Level Positive Airway Pressure) remedy is often

recommended for those who require more help for breathing beyond what a big CPAP (Continuous Positive Airway Pressure) tool can provide. BiPAP is specially appropriate for the subsequent human beings:

Respiratory Conditions: BiPAP therapy is normally prescribed for human beings with respiratory situations, along with chronic obstructive pulmonary disease (COPD), weight issues hypoventilation syndrome (OHS), or neuromuscular disorders which have an effect on breathing function. These humans frequently experience problems with respiration, in particular in the course of exhalation. The dual stress settings of BiPAP, with a better inspiratory stress (IPAP) and a decrease expiratory pressure (EPAP), can assist in improving air drift and lowering the try required to exhale.

Central Sleep Apnea: BiPAP treatment may be advocated for humans with massive sleep apnea (CSA), a state of affairs characterized with the useful resource of way of the mind's failure to deliver appropriate indicators for respiration during sleep. BiPAP gadgets with specialised algorithms can assist regulate respiration through presenting timed stress guide all through inhalation and pressure bargain at some stage in exhalation.

Complex Sleep Apnea Syndrome: Some human beings identified with complicated sleep apnea syndrome (CompSA) can also moreover require BiPAP remedy. CompSA is a aggregate of obstructive sleep apnea (OSA) and giant sleep apnea (CSA). BiPAP remedy can address every styles of apneas with the useful resource of delivering higher pressure in the course of inhalation to deal with the OSA aspect and decrease stress in some unspecified time in the future of exhalation to cope with the CSA issue.

Pressure Intolerance: Individuals who find out it tough to tolerate the everyday pressure brought by using a CPAP device may additionally additionally furthermore gain from BiPAP remedy.

BiPAP presents pressure consolation ultimately of exhalation, making it extra comfortable for people who war with exhaling in opposition to the non-save you stress.

High Pressure Requirements: Some people with sleep apnea or respiratory situations can also require higher pressure stages for effective remedy. BiPAP devices can provide the critical useful resource with the resource of way of turning in custom designed inspiratory and expiratory pressure settings.

It is vital to take a look at that the suitability of BiPAP treatment is determined based totally on man or woman wishes, sleep study effects, and the advice of a healthcare company or sleep expert. They will observe the precise breathing circumstance, severity of sleep apnea, and everyday health to determine the maximum suitable remedy technique.

three.Five Advantages and Considerations

BiPAP (Bi-Level Positive Airway Pressure) remedy offers numerous blessings for human beings with sleep apnea, breathing insufficiency, and exclusive respiration-associated troubles. Understanding the benefits and problems of BiPAP treatment can assist humans make informed alternatives concerning their remedy. Here are some key advantages and problems to keep in mind:

Advantages of BiPAP Therapy:

Enhanced Comfort: BiPAP remedy gives a extra comfortable breathing enjoy compared to non-prevent extremely good airway stress (CPAP) therapy. The twin strain settings of BiPAP, with a better inspiratory high first-class airway pressure (IPAP) for the duration of inhalation and a lower expiratory top notch airway stress (EPAP) in some unspecified time inside the destiny of exhalation, make it much less complex to respire in opposition to the stress and might purpose superior consolation.

Pressure Relief: BiPAP gadgets offer pressure comfort at some point of exhalation, decreasing the strive required to breathe out inside the path of the normal stress. This function is particularly beneficial for individuals who conflict with exhaling in opposition to the non-stop stress of CPAP remedy.

Customizable Settings: BiPAP treatment allows for custom designed strain settings to fulfill person wishes.

Healthcare companies can alter the inspiratory and expiratory pressures based totally on sleep take a look at consequences, breathing situations, and patient comfort, ensuring maximum beneficial remedy efficacy.

Respiratory Conditions: BiPAP remedy is properly-relevant for human beings with respiratory conditions which encompass persistent obstructive pulmonary infection (COPD), weight issues hypoventilation syndrome (OHS), and neuromuscular problems. The dual stress settings of BiPAP can help in enhancing air flow, lowering the try required to breathe, and helping respiration function.

Considerations for BiPAP Therapy:

Prescription and Monitoring: BiPAP treatment calls for a prescription from a healthcare provider. Regular monitoring, look at-up appointments, and adjustments to pressure settings may be crucial to make sure treatment efficacy and address any problems that could rise up.

Compliance and Adaptation: Like any sleep treatment, adherence to BiPAP remedy is crucial for number one consequences. Some human beings may also furthermore require an model period to come to be comfortable with the BiPAP device and mask. Working cautiously with healthcare agencies, sleep professionals, and help agencies can help triumph over any traumatic conditions or issues associated with compliance and version.

Cost and Availability: BiPAP devices can be greater high-priced than CPAP gadgets due to their greater capabilities and talents. It is vital to recall the price and availability of BiPAP remedy, which embody insurance coverage and capability out-of-pocket costs.

Chapter 4: Auto-Titrating Continuous Positive Airway Pressure

four.1 What is AutoCPAP?

AutoCPAP, additionally called Auto-Adjusting CPAP or APAP (Auto

Adjusting Positive Airway Pressure), is a form of continuous great airway strain treatment used to deal with sleep apnea and different breathing-associated sleep problems. AutoCPAP devices are designed to automatically regulate the added air strain based totally on an individual's breathing patterns at some level in the night time.

Here's how AutoCPAP works:

Pressure Adjustment: AutoCPAP devices constantly monitor the character's respiration the usage of advanced algorithms and sensors. These algorithms take a look at the airflow and find out changes in the resistance of the airway.

Automatic Pressure Adjustments: Based on the assessment of the individual's respiratory styles, the AutoCPAP tool dynamically adjusts the air strain introduced to the airway. The tool responds in real-time to provide the minimal powerful pressure needed to maintain an open airway in the end of sleep.

Personalized Therapy: AutoCPAP treatment offers personalised treatment by the use of way of adapting to the individual's converting wishes. It can reply to variations within the severity of sleep apnea activities, positional modifications inside the path of sleep, and different factors that may impact the airway's resistance.

Sleep Study Data: The preliminary pressure range for AutoCPAP treatment is generally determined through a snooze examine or a CPAP titration test. The sleep examine offers valuable facts about the character's sleep styles, apnea activities, and vital pressure stages. This data lets in set up a starting variety for the AutoCPAP device.

Benefits of AutoCPAP Therapy:

Customized Treatment: AutoCPAP devices offer individualized treatment with the useful resource of turning in the right stress levels wanted at any given moment. This can optimize treatment efficacy and comfort.

Adaptability: AutoCPAP devices can regulate the stress based on changes in the person's sleep position, sleep degree, or other elements that would have an impact on respiratory. This adaptability makes AutoCPAP in particular suitable for people with diverse pressure necessities at a few stage within the night time.

Ease of Use: AutoCPAP devices are customer-first-rate, as they put off the want for manual stress changes. Users can clearly positioned at the mask and allow the tool automatically modify the stress as preferred.

Compliance Monitoring: Many AutoCPAP devices have protected data recording capabilities that song treatment compliance, apnea activities, and unique parameters. This facts can be beneficial for healthcare carriers to reveal treatment improvement and make changes if important.

AutoCPAP remedy offers the advantage of offering custom designed and adaptable remedy for human beings with sleep apnea. However, it's far crucial to talk over with a healthcare company or sleep professional to decide if AutoCPAP is the maximum suitable treatment alternative based totally on character dreams, sleep have a take a look at consequences, and one of a type factors. Regular observe-up appointments are also encouraged to evaluate treatment efficacy and make any important changes.

4.2 How AutoCPAP Devices Work

AutoCPAP (Auto-Adjusting Positive Airway Pressure) gadgets, moreover referred to as APAP (Auto-Adjusting CPAP) gadgets, are

superior respiration treatment devices used within the treatment of sleep apnea and other respiratory-associated troubles. AutoCPAP devices art work through using mechanically adjusting the added air stress primarily based on the individual's breathing styles in the path of the night time time. Here's how AutoCPAP devices paintings:

Continuous Monitoring: AutoCPAP gadgets encompass advanced algorithms and sensors that constantly monitor the person's respiratory patterns. These devices can find out changes in airflow, resistance, and incredible parameters related to the airway's patency.

Pressure Adjustment: Based at the non-prevent monitoring and analysis of the character's respiratory, the AutoCPAP device dynamically adjusts the air pressure introduced to the airway.

It ambitions to offer the minimum powerful pressure required to hold an open airway and effectively address sleep apnea sports.

Real-Time Responsiveness: The AutoCPAP device responds in real-time to the character's respiration patterns. If a partial or whole airway obstruction is detected, the tool will boom the pressure to guide the airway and restore regular respiration. If the airway obstruction resolves or the resistance decreases, the tool can lessen the stress to a more snug diploma.

Algorithmic Intelligence: AutoCPAP gadgets utilize state-of-the-art algorithms that take a look at the records collected from the sensors. These algorithms don't forget different factors along with loud night breathing, go with the drift limitations, apnea activities, and adjustments in sleep characteristic. By thinking about the ones parameters, the device must make particular stress changes inside the route of the night time time time.

Data Recording and Analysis: Many AutoCPAP gadgets have incorporated facts recording capabilities. These devices can gather records on treatment compliance, apnea events, stress levels, and distinct parameters. This records may be valuable for healthcare organizations to assess remedy effectiveness, make adjustments, and screen prolonged-time period improvement.

The key gain of AutoCPAP remedy is its capacity to offer customized and adaptable treatment based totally totally at the individual's particular dreams and the dynamic nature of sleep apnea. By routinely adjusting the pressure to address adjustments within the airway's resistance, AutoCPAP devices optimize remedy efficacy and comfort.

It is important to be conscious that AutoCPAP treatment though requires a prescription from a healthcare issuer. The appropriate stress variety for the AutoCPAP tool is normally determined based on sleep have a look at results or a CPAP titration have a check. Regular follow-up appointments with healthcare corporations are advocated to display treatment improvement, examine statistics, and make any vital modifications to the stress settings or remedy technique.

four.Three Benefits of AutoCPAP Devices

AutoCPAP (Auto-Adjusting Positive Airway Pressure) devices

provide numerous advantages for people with sleep apnea and exceptional breathing-associated issues. These superior gadgets routinely alter the delivered air pressure based totally at the character's respiration patterns at some stage in the night time time. Here are some key blessings of AutoCPAP gadgets:

Personalized Treatment: One of the full-size blessings of AutoCPAP remedy is its functionality to provide custom designed remedy. The devices continuously display the character's breathing patterns and adjust the air strain therefore. This guarantees that the very satisfactory first-class pressure is delivered at any given 2d, addressing the unique dreams of the character.

Optimal Pressure Delivery: AutoCPAP devices dynamically alter the stress tiers based totally mostly on changes in the airway's resistance and the severity of sleep apnea sports activities. By imparting the proper quantity of stress had to maintain the airway open, AutoCPAP remedy can efficaciously reduce or dispose of apneas, hypopneas, and snoring.

Comfort and Adaptability: AutoCPAP gadgets provide improved consolation and versatility as compared to standard CPAP devices. The functionality to routinely alter the stress for the duration of the night time lets in people discover the maximum cushty and powerful pressure settings for his or her dreams. This can beautify standard remedy compliance and affected character pleasure.

Response to Changes: AutoCPAP gadgets can come upon adjustments in the individual's sleep role, sleep degree, or different elements that might have an effect on respiratory. The gadgets can then respond with the aid of solving the stress levels in real-time. This adaptability lets in for best treatment efficacy even in various sleep situations.

Data Recording and Analysis: Many AutoCPAP gadgets have built-in statistics recording talents, that could provide treasured insights into treatment effectiveness. The recorded facts can encompass information approximately compliance, apnea occasions, strain levels, and different parameters. Healthcare carriers can use this facts to assess the individual's improvement, make critical adjustments, and optimize the treatment over the years.

Simplified Pressure Titration: AutoCPAP devices can simplify the stress titration way. Rather than undergoing a separate sleep have a look at or titration take a look at to determine the first-rate stress settings, the tool can routinely alter the stress ranges primarily based on actual-time records. This can keep time and assets for every the person and healthcare agencies.

AutoCPAP treatment offers individualized remedy, adaptability, and comfort for people with sleep apnea.

However, it's miles important to visit a healthcare company or sleep professional to decide if AutoCPAP is the most appropriate treatment choice based totally on character wishes, sleep have a look at consequences, and various factors. Regular observe-up appointments are also recommended to assess treatment efficacy and make any essential modifications.

4.Four Adjusting Pressure Automatically

Adjusting pressure mechanically is a key function of AutoCPAP

(Auto-Adjusting Positive Airway Pressure) devices, which can be used inside the treatment of sleep apnea and different respiration-associated problems. These gadgets employ superior algorithms and sensors to constantly display the man or woman's respiration patterns and regulate the introduced air stress for this reason. Here's how the manner of solving strain robotically works:

Continuous Monitoring: AutoCPAP devices constantly display screen the character's respiratory through analyzing parameters together with airflow, go along with the float limitations, loud night breathing, and changes in resistance. The sensors embedded inside the device come across those versions at some point of the night time.

Algorithmic Analysis: The accumulated records is processed thru contemporary algorithms which might be programmed into the AutoCPAP tool. These algorithms analyze the information and locate any abnormalities or disruptions in breathing patterns, which encompass apneas or hypopneas.

Pressure Adjustment: Based at the analysis of the breathing patterns, the AutoCPAP tool robotically adjusts the air strain introduced to the airway. If it detects a partial or whole airway obstruction, the tool will boom the strain to aid the airway and promote everyday breathing. Conversely, if the airway obstruction resolves or the resistance decreases, the device reduces the stress to a extra comfortable level.

Real-Time Responsiveness: The adjustment of pressure takes vicinity in actual-time, allowing the AutoCPAP tool to answer rapidly to changes in respiration styles.

This ensures that the device offers the right pressure preferred at any given second, optimizing remedy efficacy and comfort.

Individualized Treatment: The automated strain adjustment function of AutoCPAP gadgets permits for individualized remedy. Each individual has specific respiratory styles and varying levels of airway resistance in the course of the night time time. The device adapts to the ones variations, offering customized treatment tailored to the individual's unique wishes.

The automated adjustment of pressure in AutoCPAP gadgets is aimed closer to preserving an open and unobstructed airway within the route of sleep. By continuously tracking and responding to adjustments within the character's respiratory styles, these gadgets optimize treatment effectiveness and improve sleep first-rate.

It's crucial to look at that the preliminary pressure variety for AutoCPAP remedy is commonly determined via a sleep have a take a look at or a CPAP titration look at. Healthcare carriers might also regulate the pressure settings based totally on the character's needs and responses to treatment over the years. Regular observe-up appointments with healthcare organizations are advocated to reveal remedy improvement, assessment records, and make any important adjustments to the pressure settings or therapy approach.

4.Five Monitoring and Data Collection Features Monitoring and statistics series skills are crucial components

of many contemporary-day CPAP (Continuous Positive Airway Pressure) and AutoCPAP (Auto-Adjusting Positive Airway Pressure) gadgets used inside the treatment of sleep apnea and unique respiratory-associated issues. These competencies permit for the gathering of treasured data concerning treatment effectiveness, compliance, and affected person development. Here's how tracking and data collection features paintings:

Data Recording: Many CPAP and AutoCPAP gadgets have incorporated facts recording abilties. These gadgets acquire and save records on diverse parameters, collectively with usage hours, stress degrees, mask leak fees, and the prevalence of apnea activities. This recorded information offers a whole evaluation of the man or woman's sleep styles and therapy adherence.

Compliance Monitoring: Monitoring abilities music the character's adherence to treatment. They document the period and consistency of CPAP or AutoCPAP device usage, helping healthcare providers look at the individual's compliance with the prescribed treatment. Compliance monitoring is in particular critical as steady and prolonged-time period usage of those gadgets is top to effective treatment.

Sleep Quality Assessment: The information accumulated with the resource of those gadgets can offer insights into the character's sleep amazing. By studying factors which consist of loud night breathing tiers, masks leak charges, and apnea sports, healthcare corporations can evaluate the effectiveness of the treatment in improving sleep patterns and not unusual sleep terrific.

Pressure Optimization: Monitoring and facts series abilties allow healthcare providers to evaluate the adequacy of strain settings. By reviewing the records recorded with the aid of the tool, healthcare vendors can observe the character's reaction to treatment, alter pressure degrees if essential, and optimize treatment effectiveness. Remote Monitoring: Some CPAP and AutoCPAP devices provide some distance flung tracking competencies.

This allows healthcare companies to remotely get proper of get admission to to the records accrued through using manner of the device and music the individual's development with out requiring in-individual visits. Remote tracking can streamline the tracking system, beautify affected person care, and allow for well timed intervention if any troubles rise up.

Treatment Adjustments: The data accumulated thru monitoring abilties allows healthcare vendors make informed alternatives regarding remedy adjustments. They can end up aware about areas which could require trade, which consist of stress settings, masks kind, or humidification settings. These adjustments can decorate remedy efficacy, decorate comfort, and cope with any troubles that may impact remedy adherence.

Chapter 5: Oral Appliances

five.1 Overview of Oral Appliances

Oral home equipment, additionally known as mandibular development gadgets (MAD) or oral sleep apnea domestic device, are dental gadgets used in the remedy of sleep apnea and snoring. These appliances are designed to be worn at some point of sleep to help preserve an open and unobstructed airway. Here's a pinnacle stage view of oral appliances:

Design and Function: Oral domestic equipment are commonly custom-made by way of dental specialists to in form the person's mouth. They are worn in addition to a sports activities sports sports mouthguard or a dental retainer. Oral home equipment artwork thru repositioning the jaw and tongue beforehand, which lets in prevent the collapse of the airway and decrease the superiority of apneas and snoring.

Types of Oral Appliances: There are one-of-a-type kinds of oral appliances to be had, along with mandibular development gadgets (MAD) and tongue-preserving devices. MADs are the most common kind and art work through advancing the lower jaw barely ahead to growth the space behind the throat. Tongue-preserving devices, alternatively, maintain the tongue in a ahead function to save you it from blockading the airway.

Customization and Fitting: Oral domestic tool are custom-made to healthful the man or woman's teeth and mouth. A dental expert takes impressions of the individual's tooth and jaw to create a customized tool. The tool is then adjusted and suited for make certain proper alignment and luxury.

Advantages of Oral Appliances: Oral home device provide numerous advantages within the remedy of sleep apnea. They are non-invasive and clean to apply, making them a more comfortable possibility to non-stop top notch airway strain (CPAP) therapy for some people. Oral appliances also are portable and convenient for excursion.

Effectiveness: Oral domestic system can be effective in decreasing the severity of sleep apnea and assuaging snoring. They assist hold an open airway via way of using repositioning the jaw and tongue.

However, the effectiveness of oral appliances can also variety counting on the individual's precise situation and the type of appliance used.

Follow-up Care: Regular follow-up visits with the dental expert are crucial to display the development of the remedy and make sure the proper healthy and characteristic of the oral device. Adjustments may be made to the device if needed to optimize its effectiveness.

Suitability: Oral home system are normally encouraged for human beings with slight to mild obstructive sleep apnea who're unable to tolerate or pick out an opportunity to CPAP remedy. They also can be suitable for human beings with positional sleep apnea or as an accessory remedy in combination with different treatment options.

It's vital to talk over with a dental expert or sleep professional to decide if an oral equipment is suitable for an character's specific desires. A thorough evaluation and assessment will help determine the maximum suitable treatment approach for sleep apnea or loud night breathing.

five.2 How Oral Appliances Treat Sleep Apnea Oral domestic equipment, additionally called mandibular development devices

(MAD) or oral sleep apnea domestic equipment, are effective remedy alternatives for human beings with slight to moderate obstructive sleep apnea (OSA). These devices paintings through repositioning the jaw and tongue forward to assist preserve an open and unobstructed airway throughout sleep. Here's how oral domestic tool deal with sleep apnea:

Airway Opening: Oral home equipment artwork with the aid of repositioning the decrease jaw (mandible) slightly forward. This forward movement allows pull the tongue and clean tissues far from the once more of the throat, thereby developing more location and stopping airway crumble or obstruction.

By keeping the airway open, oral home machine lessen the occurrence of apneas (pauses in breathing) and decorate oxygen waft for the duration of sleep. Reduction in Snoring: Snoring is a common symptom of sleep apnea. Oral domestic system assist alleviate snoring through using repositioning the jaw and tongue, which lets in to lessen the vibration of mild tissues inside the throat that reasons loud night breathing. This not handiest improves sleep high-quality for the person however moreover benefits their sleep partner.

Customized Fit: Oral home device are custom-made to suit every man or woman's mouth and enamel. Dental experts take impressions of the man or woman's enamel and jaw to create a custom designed tool that offers finest comfort and effectiveness. The custom designed in form ensures that the device is secure discomfort or infection.

and does no longer reason

Non-Invasive Treatment: Oral home device provide a non-invasive

treatment alternative for sleep apnea. Unlike non-prevent notable airway pressure (CPAP) therapy, which includes wearing a mask and delivering pressurized air, oral home equipment are more snug and less intrusive. This can enhance remedy compliance and beautify commonplace affected person pleasure.

Portability and Convenience: Oral home system are transportable and on hand for excursion.

They are small, lightweight, and easy to maintain, making them an attractive possibility for individuals who frequently excursion or have an active lifestyle.

The comfort of oral domestic gadget encourages everyday usage, that is crucial for powerful treatment.

Adjunct to Other Treatments: Oral home device additionally may be used as an accessory remedy in combination with brilliant treatment options. For folks that locate it difficult to tolerate CPAP remedy, oral domestic equipment can offer a likely opportunity or be carried out in combination with CPAP to beautify remedy consequences.

It is critical to speak about with a dental expert or sleep expert to decide if an oral equipment is appropriate for an person's unique goals. A thorough evaluation, which incorporates a sleep have a examine, will help decide the severity of sleep apnea and the maximum appropriate treatment method. Regular comply with-up visits with the dental professional are essential to show remedy effectiveness and make any essential modifications to the oral equipment.

five.Three Types of Oral Appliances

There are several varieties of oral appliances, moreover called mandibular improvement devices (MAD), used inside the treatment of sleep apnea and snoring. These devices are designed to be worn within the direction of sleep and paintings with the aid of the usage of repositioning the jaw and tongue to assist preserve an open and unobstructed airway. Here are some common styles of oral appliances:

Mandibular Advancement Devices (MADs): MADs are the most usually used sort of oral domestic gadget for sleep apnea. They consist of two separate trays that healthy over the higher and lower enamel, related with the aid of hinges. By adjusting the hinge and shifting the decrease jaw in advance, MADs assist reposition the tongue and moderate tissues to prevent airway fall apart and enhance airflow.

Tongue-Retaining Devices: Tongue-maintaining gadgets are designed to hold the tongue in a earlier function all through sleep.

These home equipment have a small compartment that suits at some stage in the tongue and a suction bulb that continues the tongue in area. By stopping the tongue from blocking off the airway, tongue-maintaining devices assist preserve an open and unobstructed airflow.

Hybrid Oral Appliances: Hybrid oral appliances integrate capabilities of each MADs and tongue-retaining gadgets. These devices embody mechanisms to broaden the lower jaw and now have a thing to maintain the tongue in a beforehand function. The mixture of those talents helps enhance the airway's patency and decrease the prevalence of sleep apnea activities.

Adjustable Oral Appliances: Adjustable oral home gadget permit for first-class-tuning of the lower jaw position. These gadgets have mechanisms that may be adjusted to regularly raise the lower jaw in small increments.

This adjustability allows for individualized remedy and excellent consolation.

Customized Fit Appliances: Many oral home device are custommade through the usage of dental professionals to ensure a selected and snug match. These appliances are designed primarily based mostly on the person's dental impressions and precise oral characteristics. Customization allows decorate effectiveness and luxury, as the equipment is tailored to the man or woman's mouth.

It's essential to talk over with a dental expert or sleep expert to determine the most suitable form of oral tool based certainly on the character's specific dreams and state of affairs. A thorough assessment, along with an assessment of the person's sleep apnea severity, jaw shape, and dental health, will help determine the maximum suitable type of oral device. Regular take a look at-up visits with the dental expert are crucial to show remedy improvement and make any crucial adjustments to make certain maximum appropriate treatment efficacy.

5.Four Benefits and Considerations

Oral domestic system, furthermore called mandibular advancement devices

(MAD), offer severa blessings as a treatment option for sleep apnea and loud night breathing. These devices artwork via repositioning the jaw and tongue to help hold an open and unobstructed airway within the course of sleep. However, it's miles important to don't forget every the benefits and worries earlier than selecting oral gadget treatment. Here are some key elements to maintain in mind:

Benefits of Oral Appliances:

Non-Invasive: Oral home equipment provide a non-invasive treatment alternative for sleep apnea. They do not require surgical treatment or the usage of masks or tubing like wonderful treatment techniques. This may want to lead them to a more snug and reachable desire for individuals who are unable to tolerate or choose out an opportunity to continuous effective airway pressure (CPAP) treatment.

Improved Sleep Quality: Oral domestic equipment can effectively lessen or do away with snoring and enhance sleep exquisite for people with sleep apnea. By keeping an open airway and stopping airway collapse, those gadgets assist make certain uninterrupted respiratory and higher oxygen flow for the duration of sleep.

Portability and Convenience: Oral domestic system are portable and smooth to use.

They are compact, mild-weight, and do not require energy, making them to be had for travel or use out of doors the house. Their portability encourages regular utilization, this is critical for effective treatment.

Comfortable Alternative: For individuals who find CPAP remedy uncomfortable or revel in masks-related problems, oral home system can provide a greater cushty opportunity. The custom-made format and adjustable match assist ensure most tremendous comfort and reduce the possibility of pain or irritation.

Considerations for Oral Appliance Therapy:

Efficacy: While oral home equipment are effective for masses humans with moderate to mild sleep apnea, they will not be appropriate for everyone. The effectiveness of oral domestic gadget can variety relying on the character's specific situation, anatomy, and the severity of sleep apnea.

It's essential to talk over with a dental professional or sleep professional to determine if an oral equipment is appropriate for a specific case.

Customization   customization   and Maintenance: Oral appliances require

and regular observe-up visits with a dental professional. The tool desires to be well equipped and modified to make certain best effectiveness and comfort.

Additionally, oral hygiene and maintenance of the machine are important to keep away from any dental troubles or headaches.

Jaw Discomfort or Bite Changes: Some human beings might also additionally enjoy brief jaw pain or chunk changes on the same time as the usage of oral domestic gadget. These thing outcomes typically subside through the years, however it's far vital to show any modifications and talk them with the dental expert.

Compliance and Monitoring: adherence to oral equipment

Like any sleep apnea remedy, remedy is essential for gold standard effects. Regular observe-up visits and monitoring by using a dental expert are critical to evaluate remedy effectiveness, make any critical changes, and make sure long-term compliance.

It's important to speak about with a dental expert or sleep expert to decide if oral appliance remedy is suitable for an man or woman's unique dreams. A thorough assessment will assist determine the severity of sleep apnea, the individual's anatomy, and the maximum suitable treatment method.

Regular take a look at-up appointments and open conversation with healthcare organizations are key to accomplishing the satisfactory outcomes with oral device remedy.

five.Five Choosing the Right Oral Appliance

Choosing the proper oral equipment for the remedy of sleep apnea or loud night breathing is important to make sure top of the line effectiveness and comfort. With various alternatives available, it is important to go through in thoughts severa elements whilst choosing an oral machine. Here are some key factors to do not forget at the same time as deciding on the right oral device:

Diagnosis and Severity: Consult with a dental professional or sleep professional to determine the right analysis and severity of sleep apnea or snoring. The severity of the situation and the individual's unique desires will help manual the selection of the most appropriate oral device.

Professional Evaluation: Seek steerage from a dental expert professional in dental sleep medication. They can perform a complete evaluation of your oral health, jaw shape, and other factors to determine the maximum appropriate shape of oral equipment on your unique desires.

Customization: Consider a custom-made oral system this is tailored to suit your mouth and enamel. Customization ensures a very specific match and most suitable consolation. A dental professional will take impressions of your enamel and jaw to create a personalized device that meets your specific requirements.

Type of Oral Appliance: There are unique styles of oral home machine to be had, which includes mandibular improvement devices (MADs) and tongue-maintaining gadgets.

Chapter 6: Positional Therapy Devices

6.1 Understanding Positional Therapy

Positional treatment is a non-invasive treatment approach used to manipulate positional obstructive sleep apnea (POSA) or positionrelated loud night breathing. It consists of changing the slumbering function to lessen or eliminate the prevalence of apneas and enhance respiration sooner or later of sleep. Understanding positional remedy can help human beings optimize their sleep feature for higher sleep super and decreased symptoms. Here's an define of positional remedy:

Positional Obstructive Sleep Apnea (POSA): POSA refers to sleep apnea that predominantly occurs while an person is sound asleep in wonderful positions, together with supine (at the another time). The airway turns into extra at risk of crumble or obstruction in the ones positions, primary to respiratory interruptions and sleep disturbances.

Changing Sleep Position: Positional remedy objectives to encourage individuals to sleep in positions that promote better airway patency and decrease the prevalence of apneas. For POSA, the primary reason is to avoid the supine function and sleep on the aspect (lateral feature) or stomach (willing function).

Positional Aids and Devices: Various aids and gadgets can assist people in keeping a specific sleep function. These can embody particularly designed pillows, positional belts or backpacks, and gadgets that provide positional remarks, which include vibration or sound, to alert the individual in the occasion that they shift right right into a supine function subsequently of sleep.

Efficacy: Positional remedy can be powerful for people with POSA who experience apneas predominantly in the supine position. By averting the supine function, people can appreciably lessen the frequency and severity of apneas. However, it's far crucial to word that positional treatment might not be powerful for human beings with sleep apnea that takes location no matter sleep feature or for people with excessive sleep apnea.

Combination Therapy: Positional treatment may be used on my own or in combination with specific treatment strategies, along with non-prevent brilliant airway pressure (CPAP) or oral domestic gadget.

In some times, people also can require options to efficaciously manipulate sleep apnea. Extra remedy Lifestyle Adjustments: In addition to positional treatment,

people may additionally gain from life-style changes. These can consist of weight manipulate, ordinary exercise, warding off alcohol and sedatives earlier than bedtime, and maintaining a consistent sleep time table.

It's critical to consult professional to determine with a healthcare business enterprise or sleep

if positional therapy is appropriate for managing sleep apnea or snoring. They can investigate the precise needs and circumstance of the character and advocate appropriate remedy techniques. Regular observe-up visits are crucial to show screen the effectiveness of positional treatment and make any important adjustments or changes to the remedy plan.

6.2 How Positional Therapy Devices Work

Positional therapy devices are designed to assist humans

hold a particular sleep role that promotes higher airway patency and decreases the prevalence of positional obstructive sleep apnea (POSA) or position-associated loud night breathing. These devices purpose to inspire individuals to keep away from snoozing in positions that make contributions to airway crumble or obstruction. Here's how positional remedy devices work:

Positional Feedback Devices: These devices use severa mechanisms to provide comments while an person shifts right right into a supine feature within the direction of sleep. They are normally worn or located at the frame and can come across modifications in sleep function.

Examples of positional feedback devices embody vibrating gadgets, sound alarms, or wearable sensors.

Vibrating Devices: These devices are worn on the body, along aspect across the waist or chest, and provide vibration cues at the same time as the person starts offevolved offevolved to sleep within the supine position. The vibration serves as a mild reminder to spark off the character to exchange their sleep function.

Sound Alarms: Sound alarm gadgets are placed near the bed and use sound cues to alert the man or woman within the occasion that they shift into the supine function. The sound alarm can be custom designed based totally at the man or woman's preference and sensitivity.

Wearable Sensors: These devices are worn at the frame or included right right into a wearable device, which includes a wristband or smartwatch. They use motion sensors to discover sleep characteristic adjustments and offer remarks, which includes vibration or auditory cues, to inspire the individual to change their sleep characteristic.

Positional Pillows and Supports: Positional treatment gadgets furthermore embody mainly designed pillows or allows that encourage people to sleep on their factor or stomach. These pillows have specific shapes or contours that assist align the frame in a preferred sleep function, lowering the danger of sound asleep on the decrease back. Side-Sleeping Pillows: These pillows have a format that helps the pinnacle, neck, and shoulders while drowsing on the aspect. They provide cushioning and right alignment to keep a lateral sleep feature.

Wedge Pillows: Wedge pillows have an inclined layout that encourages people to sleep on their side or at an mind-set. The incline facilitates reduce the tendency to sleep at the again and promotes better airflow.

Body Positioners: Body positioners are foam or inflatable gadgets that offer manual to maintain the frame in a specific sleep feature. They may be placed maximum of the legs or at some stage in the torso to prevent rolling onto the once more.

Positional remedy devices artwork through imparting cues, reminders, or physical assist to inspire humans to sleep in positions that limit airway obstruction. These gadgets can be used by myself or in aggregate with different treatment options, including non-stop quality airway strain (CPAP) or oral domestic equipment, counting on the severity and person desires. It's crucial to talk approximately with a healthcare organisation or sleep professional to determine the most appropriate positional therapy device for handling POSA or loud night breathing and to make sure right usage and effectiveness.

6.3 Types of Positional Therapy Devices

Positional treatment devices are designed to assist people keep a selected sleep characteristic that promotes better airway patency and decreases positional obstructive sleep apnea (POSA) or function-related loud night breathing. These gadgets can be powerful in encouraging human beings to avoid napping on their again, this is regularly associated with airway crumble or obstruction. Here are a few common types of positional therapy gadgets:

Positional Feedback Devices: These devices provide remarks when an person shifts right proper right into a supine function all through sleep. They can use numerous mechanisms to alert the man or woman, together with vibrations, sounds, or alarms. Examples encompass:

Wearable Sensors: These gadgets are normally worn on the frame, which incorporates on the chest or wrist, and use motion sensors to discover sleep function adjustments. When the person starts offevolved to sleep on their again, the tool can provide slight vibrations or auditory cues to set off them to shift to a facet or stomach role.

Ball-in-Socket Devices: These devices are placed in a small pouch connected to the again of the sleepwear. The ball rolls or movements on the equal time because the individual is in a supine characteristic, imparting sensory comments to inspire changing positions.

Positional Pillows and Supports: These in particular designed pillows and helps help human beings preserve a lateral (issue) or inclined (belly) sleep function, lowering the chance of dozing at the decrease lower back. Examples consist of:

Wedge Pillows: Wedge-normal pillows have an incline that discourages slumbering on the lower back and promotes aspect-napping. The incline lets in preserve higher airway alignment and respiration eventually of sleep.

Body Positioners: These gadgets are positioned most of the legs or across the torso to offer guide and inspire side-napping. Body positioners may be made from foam, inflatable materials, or adjustable straps.

Tennis Ball Technique: This smooth method consists of sewing a tennis ball onto the once more of sleepwear or placing it in a pocket on the once more. The ache due to the tennis ball encourages the person to shift to a aspect-sleeping function.

Bed Positioning Devices: These gadgets are used to modify the overall positioning of the mattress to promote lateral sleep positions. Examples include:

Inclined Sleep Systems: These structures improve the upper body or the entire bed at an incline, making it more comfortable and herbal to sleep at the issue.

Lateral Sleep Trainers: These devices characteristic a cushioned barrier at the element of the mattress to bodily prevent the person from rolling onto their lower back throughout sleep.

The choice of positional treatment device is based totally upon on factors which encompass personal preference, consolation, and effectiveness. It is critical to talk over with a healthcare provider or sleep expert to decide the most appropriate tool for handling POSA or snoring, considering person needs and sleep patterns. Regular study-up visits can help show development and make any critical modifications to optimize treatment efficacy.

6.Four Effectiveness and Considerations

Positional remedy gadgets are designed to assist humans

maintain a selected sleep feature that promotes better airflow and decreases the prevalence of positional obstructive sleep apnea (POSA) or characteristic-related snoring. While those gadgets can be effective for plenty human beings, it is important to undergo in thoughts their effectiveness and high-quality concerns whilst the usage of them. Here's an outline:

Effectiveness of Positional Therapy Devices:

POSA Management: Positional remedy devices may be significantly powerful in coping with POSA.

By encouraging human beings to sleep in positions aside from supine (at the yet again), those gadgets help lower airway fall apart and obstruction, decreasing the frequency and severity of apneas. They can notably improve sleep best and common nicely-being.

Snoring Reduction: Position-associated snoring additionally may be successfully addressed with positional remedy gadgets. By promoting facet or stomach sleeping positions, the ones devices help keep the airway open and reduce the vibration of easy tissues, thereby lowering or eliminating snoring.

Individual Variation: The effectiveness of positional remedy gadgets can vary among humans. Some people also can experience big development in sleep apnea or loud night breathing symptoms and signs and symptoms, whilst others can also see more modest effects. The effectiveness may additionally moreover rely upon factors together with the underlying motive of sleep apnea, body habitus, severity of the scenario, and adherence to treatment.

Considerations for Positional Therapy Devices:

Sleep Position Compliance: The success of positional remedy is based at the man or woman's functionality to continually hold the popular sleep role sooner or later of the night time time. It may additionally additionally take time to regulate and increase a addiction of drowsing within the endorsed function, especially for humans familiar with supine snoozing. Compliance with positional remedy is crucial for remaining effectiveness.

Individual Suitability: Not every body with sleep apnea or snoring are appropriate applicants for positional remedy devices. The effectiveness of those devices on the whole relies upon on the connection between sleep feature and airway collapse. Individuals with sleep apnea that takes place regardless of sleep function or with excessive sleep apnea might not benefit as an entire lot from positional remedy by myself.

Combination Therapy: Positional treatment devices can be used as standalone remedy alternatives or in combination with wonderful remedies, which include non-prevent high-quality airway pressure (CPAP) or oral home machine. Combination treatment may be extra powerful for people with extra extreme sleep apnea or those who experience apneas in multiple sleep positions.

Professional Guidance: It is clearly beneficial to visit a healthcare organization or sleep expert earlier than the use of positional treatment gadgets. They can observe the man or woman's scenario, check the suitability of positional remedy, and offer steering on the appropriate tool and utilization.

Personal Comfort: Each person can also additionally have distinctive options and luxury ranges with numerous positional treatment gadgets. Finding the device this is maximum snug and conducive to retaining the popular sleep feature is essential for long-time period adherence and effectiveness.

Positional treatment gadgets may be treasured equipment in handling POSA and characteristic-associated snoring. However, it's far crucial to speak over with a healthcare issuer or sleep professional to determine the most appropriate therapy approach based on character needs and situations. Regular have a look at-up visits are crucial to show development and make any critical modifications to optimize treatment effectiveness.

6.Five Combining Positional Therapy with Other Treatments

Combining positional remedy with other remedies can be a useful approach in coping with sleep apnea, in particular even as

positional obstructive sleep apnea (POSA) or characteristic-related loud night breathing is a

modalities

contributing element. By using a couple of remedy

simultaneously, human beings can optimize the effectiveness of treatment and enhance sleep satisfactory. Here are a few key issues and blessings of blending positional remedy with different treatments:

Continuous Positive Airway Pressure (CPAP): CPAP therapy is a commonly used treatment for sleep apnea.

When combining positional treatment with CPAP, humans can benefit from both interventions. Using positional remedy gadgets, which incorporates positional pillows or feedback gadgets, can help inspire dozing in non-supine positions, that may beautify CPAP treatment efficacy via lowering airway obstruction and improving compliance.

Oral Appliance Therapy: Oral appliances, alongside side mandibular development devices (MADs), are some other remedy preference for sleep apnea. Combining positional treatment with oral device remedy may be specifically useful for individuals who've positional factors to their sleep apnea. Positional therapy can help further enhance airflow with the resource of using encouraging the protection of a lateral or susceptible sleep function at the identical time as carrying the oral system.

Weight Management: Weight loss can extensively decorate sleep apnea signs and signs and symptoms in folks which might be overweight or overweight.

Combining positional remedy with weight manipulate strategies, which embody a healthful weight loss plan and ordinary workout, can in addition beautify the effectiveness of remedy. By addressing each positional factors and weight loss, individuals might also moreover revel in superior airway patency and reduced sleep apnea severity.

Lifestyle Modifications: Incorporating lifestyle changes can manual the effectiveness of positional treatment.

Chapter 7: Adaptive Servo-Ventilation

7.1 What is ASV?

ASV stands for Adaptive Servo-Ventilation. It is a specialized shape of effective airway stress treatment used in the remedy of positive sleep-disordered breathing situations, in particular applicable sleep apnea (CSA) and complicated sleep apnea syndrome (CompSA). ASV devices supply variable strain assist to make certain adequate air glide and keep a solid respiratory pattern at some point of sleep.

ASV works via way of manner of continuously monitoring the person's respiratory sample and adjusting the brought stress help primarily based absolutely mostly on the detected respiration events. It uses a mixture of inspiratory extremely good airway pressure (IPAP) and expiratory powerful airway strain (EPAP) to assist and optimize ventilation. The tool automatically adjusts the stress ranges on a breath-by way of-breath foundation, responding to adjustments in breathing attempt and adapting to the person's specific needs.

ASV remedy is mainly beneficial for human beings with CSA, wherein there's a disruption within the mind's control of respiration at some point of sleep. It additionally can be useful for people with CompSA, a circumstance characterised thru a combination of obstructive and primary sleep apnea sports.

ASV treatment ambitions to stabilize the breathing pattern, normalize air flow, and reduce the frequency of apneas and hypopneas inside the direction of sleep. By supplying adaptive strain useful resource, it enables make certain suitable sufficient airflow, oxygenation, and air waft, ensuing in stepped forward sleep exceptional, decreased daylight sleepiness, and better everyday respiratory function.

It's crucial to notice that ASV remedy want to be prescribed and monitored thru a healthcare expert focusing on sleep medicine.

They will decide if ASV is the best remedy opportunity primarily based definitely virtually on the character's specific assessment, sleep observe consequences, and everyday health. Regular observe-up visits and changes are critical to make certain the remedy remains powerful and to address any potential problems.

7.2 How ASV Devices Work

ASV (Adaptive Servo-Ventilation) gadgets are superior excellent airway stress devices used in the remedy of sleep-disordered

respiratory situations, specially crucial sleep apnea (CSA) and complicated sleep apnea syndrome (CompSA).

These gadgets artwork through delivering variable strain assist to ensure ok air go along with the go with the flow and stabilize the breathing sample throughout sleep. Here's how ASV gadgets artwork:

Monitoring Respiratory Pattern: ASV devices constantly

display screen the character's respiratory sample at some degree inside the night time. They use modern-day sensors and algorithms to hit upon adjustments in respiration try and the occurrence of apneas, hypopneas, or other respiratory irregularities.

Variable Pressure Support: Based on the real-time tracking of breathing occasions, ASV gadgets routinely alter the introduced strain assist to optimize ventilation. They supply inspiratory pleasant airway strain (IPAP) to assist with inhalation and expiratory superb airway pressure (EPAP) to keep an open airway within the course of exhalation.

Adaptive Algorithm: ASV devices appoint an adaptive set of rules that analyzes the person's respiratory sample and dynamically adjusts the pressure degrees on a breath-by way of the usage of-breath foundation. The set of rules responds to modifications in respiration attempt, adjusting the stress resource to satisfy the character's unique dreams for the duration of the night time time.

Pressure Oscillation: ASV gadgets regularly include strain oscillation, which incorporates unexpectedly fluctuating the added pressure within a prescribed range. This oscillation allows hold airway patency, smooth any obstruction, and stimulate the breathing system to build up greater everyday respiration styles.

Optimal Ventilation: By presenting variable stress manual, ASV gadgets goal to stabilize the breathing sample and ensure maximum beneficial air glide. They assist keep a ordinary and normal respiratory price, decrease the occurrence of number one apneas or hypopneas, and enhance the change of oxygen and carbon dioxide at some point of sleep.

Data Collection: ASV devices commonly have statistics recording skills that acquire and keep facts approximately the man or woman's breathing styles, compliance, and treatment efficacy. This records can be useful for healthcare groups to assess remedy effectiveness, make adjustments if needed, and display the person's development over the years.

ASV devices are prescribed and monitored via healthcare experts specialized in sleep remedy. They determine if ASV remedy is suitable primarily based absolutely at the character's particular analysis, sleep have a examine effects, and common fitness. Regular followup visits are essential to assess remedy effectiveness, make any vital adjustments, and ensure pinnacle of the line treatment consequences.

7.Three Indications for ASV Therapy

ASV (Adaptive Servo-Ventilation) treatment is a specialised form of

amazing airway stress remedy used within the treatment of sure sleep-disordered breathing conditions. It is on the complete indicated for human beings who've vital sleep apnea (CSA) or complicated sleep apnea syndrome (CompSA). Here are the symptoms for ASV remedy:

Central Sleep Apnea (CSA): ASV treatment is generally used for humans with CSA, a form of sleep apnea characterized through the mind's failure to transmit suitable indicators to the respiration muscle tissues, resulting in a loss of breathing try at some stage in sleep. ASV remedy enables stabilize the respiratory sample and repair normal air flow with the resource of turning in variable pressure help.

Complex Sleep Apnea Syndrome (CompSA): CompSA refers to a situation wherein people first of all have obstructive sleep apnea (OSA) but increase valuable apneas even as treated with non-save you first-class airway pressure (CPAP). ASV remedy is considered an effective remedy for CompSA as it is able to address every the obstructive and crucial components of the sleep apnea occasions.

Inadequate Response to Other Therapies: ASV remedy can be indicated for individuals who have no longer spoke back nicely to distinct treatment modalities along with CPAP, bilevel high-quality airway strain (BiPAP), or oxygen treatment. It is especially useful even as there's a essential element of essential apneas.

Treatment of Sleep-Related Hypoventilation: ASV remedy also can be taken into consideration for people with sleep-associated hypoventilation, a circumstance wherein there's inadequate air go together with the drift at some stage in sleep ensuing in excessive levels of carbon dioxide (hypercapnia). ASV can assist optimize air go with the flow and deal with the hypoventilation related to positive respiration or neuromuscular problems.

Coexisting Cardiovascular Conditions: ASV remedy can be beneficial for individuals with CSA and coexisting cardiovascular conditions collectively with coronary heart failure with reduced ejection fraction. It can help improve respiration patterns and air drift, lowering the load on the cardiovascular machine during sleep.

It's critical to be aware that ASV remedy must be prescribed and monitored through the usage of healthcare professionals specialized in sleep medication. They will evaluate the character's precise analysis, sleep have a study outcomes, and common health to decide the high-quality treatment approach. Regular comply with-up visits and communique with the healthcare business enterprise are important to assess remedy effectiveness, make any crucial modifications, and make sure best treatment effects.

7.Four Benefits and Potential Risks

ASV (Adaptive Servo-Ventilation) remedy is a specialized form of

top notch airway pressure treatment used in the treatment of sleepdisordered respiration situations, especially valuable sleep apnea (CSA) and complex sleep apnea syndrome (CompSA). ASV treatment gives numerous benefits however moreover includes powerful ability risks. Here's a pinnacle level view:

#Benefits of ASV Therapy:

Improved Sleep Quality: ASV remedy allows stabilize the breathing pattern and optimize air flow sooner or later of sleep. By handing over variable pressure help, it reduces the frequency of vital apneas and hypopneas, main to improved sleep terrific and uninterrupted sleep.

Enhanced Oxygenation: ASV treatment supports desirable sufficient airflow and air flow, making sure superior oxygenation stages for the duration of sleep. This may additionally moreover have a super effect on normal cardiovascular health and decrease the danger of headaches related to untreated sleep apnea.

Treatment for Central Sleep Apnea: ASV treatment is notably effective in managing valuable sleep apnea, a situation characterized thru the thoughts's failure to transmit appropriate signals to the breathing muscle tissues.

It lets in repair regular ventilation and decrease the superiority of imperative apneas and sleep-associated respiration disturbances.

Treatment for Complex Sleep Apnea Syndrome: ASV treatment is indicated for humans with complicated sleep apnea syndrome (CompSA), in which there may be a aggregate of obstructive and relevant apneas. It addresses both additives of the sleep apnea activities, imparting complete treatment for this condition.

Potential Risks of ASV Therapy:

Increased Risk of Central Apnea: In some uncommon times, ASV remedy also can in all likelihood exacerbate valuable apnea sports activities. This can rise up in human beings with positive cardiac situations or excessive CSA. Close monitoring and everyday look at-up with a healthcare expert are crucial to select out and control any detrimental outcomes.

Mask Discomfort and Air Leakage: Similar to different notable airway pressure treatments, people the usage of ASV treatment may moreover revel in masks discomfort or air leakage. Proper masks fitting and adjustments are crucial to decrease these problems and enhance treatment adherence and comfort.

Adherence and Compliance Challenges: ASV treatment, like exclusive sleep apnea remedies, calls for regular usage sooner or later of the night time time to gain closing results. Some humans may additionally moreover locate it difficult to comply to the treatment or can also have difficulties tolerating the pressure settings. Ensuring suitable communication with the healthcare business enterprise, addressing any issues right away, and supplying vital aid can assist improve adherence and compliance.

Cost and Availability: ASV treatment also can contain better fees in comparison to different quality airway pressure remedy alternatives. Availability can also additionally variety depending on geographic area and healthcare assets. It is vital to talk about the ones elements with the healthcare business enterprise and coverage agency to decide the feasibility and insurance of ASV remedy.

It's critical to are trying to find advice from a healthcare professional specialised in sleep treatment to assess the suitability of ASV remedy, speak ability dangers, and examine the benefits with regards to an man or woman's specific scenario. Regular take a look at-up visits and open communication are crucial to expose treatment efficacy, cope with any worries, and make adjustments as needed to optimize treatment consequences.

7.Five Monitoring and Adjustments

Monitoring and making essential changes are essential factors of making sure the effectiveness and maximum dependable outcomes of ASV (Adaptive Servo-Ventilation) treatment.

Regular monitoring lets in healthcare experts to assess remedy efficacy, study adherence, and make suitable adjustments to address any issues which could upward push up all through the path of remedy. Here's a pinnacle degree view of tracking and modifications in ASV remedy:

Initial Assessment: Before whole evaluation is beginning ASV treatment, a

done through a healthcare professional specializing in sleep medicinal drug. This assessment consists of an extensive clinical facts, physical examination, sleep have a look at results, and evaluation of the person's unique sleepdisordered respiration situation. It permits determine the amazing ASV device settings and treatment parameters.

Titration Study: A titration test is regularly achieved to splendid-music the ASV tool settings and optimize treatment. This look at is usually completed in a nap laboratory under the supervision of sleep experts. It involves tracking the individual's sleep and respiratory patterns while adjusting the strain ranges and one-of-a-type parameters of the ASV device to achieve most beneficial air drift and remedy efficacy.

Compliance Monitoring: Regular comply with-up visits are scheduled to reveal the man or woman's compliance with ASV treatment. Compliance facts, including utilization hours and adherence to treatment, can be downloaded from the ASV tool and reviewed through healthcare professionals. This information allows decide treatment adherence and grow to be aware about any capability problems that may effect treatment effectiveness.

Data Analysis: ASV therapy gadgets often have built-in data collection abilties that file relevant data, on the facet of apnea-hypopnea index (AHI), leak costs, and breathing activities. Sleep specialists and healthcare vendors can analyze this records to evaluate remedy efficacy, pick out tendencies, and make critical adjustments to optimize treatment consequences.

Adjustments and Fine-Tuning: Based at the facts analysis and character feedback, healthcare specialists might also want to make adjustments to the ASV device settings, which include stress useful resource, EPAP, and one-of-a-kind parameters. These adjustments aim to deal with any troubles or optimize remedy based totally mostly on the man or woman's response, adherence, and remedy goals.

Chapter 8: Surgical Options For Sleep Apnea

eight.1 Overview of Surgical Treatments

Surgical treatments for sleep apnea are commonly considered even as awesome conservative remedy alternatives, collectively with first-class airway strain treatment or oral domestic system, have no longer provided awesome outcomes or aren't suitable for an individual. These surgical interventions purpose to address the underlying anatomical or structural abnormalities that make contributions to sleep apnea. Here's an outline of a few not unusual surgical remedies for sleep apnea:

Uvulopalatopharyngoplasty (UPPP): UPPP is one of the maximum not unusual surgical strategies for sleep apnea. The uvula, tonsils, and part of the soft palate are the various more tissue in the throat that want to be eliminated. UPPP goals to widen the airway and reduce obstructions that make a contribution to sleep apnea.

Maxillomandibular Advancement (MMA): MMA is a system that repositions the better and reduce jaw to boom the distance in the airway. By advancing the jaws forward, MMA enables amplify the airway and reduce the collapsibility of the clean tissues, therefore enhancing airflow at some point of sleep.

Nasal Surgery: Nasal surgical remedy may be performed to accurate nasal abnormalities or obstructions that make contributions to sleep apnea.

Procedures which incorporates septoplasty (straightening the nasal septum), turbinate reduce fee (reducing the dimensions of nasal turbinates), or nasal valve reconstruction can assist improve nasal airflow and decrease resistance.

Tongue Base Surgery: Tongue base surgical strategies, which includes genioglossus development or hyoid suspension, purpose to cope with tongue-related obstructions. These tactics reposition the tongue or anchor it to save you it from collapsing backward and obstructing the airway at some stage in sleep.

Tracheostomy: Tracheostomy is a surgical treatment that involves growing a eternal taking off in the trachea (windpipe). It is typically considered a final inn and reserved for extreme times of sleep apnea which might be unresponsive to distinct remedies. Tracheostomy bypasses the pinnacle airway in reality, allowing air to glide right now into the lungs.

It's important to word that surgical remedies for sleep apnea are usually considered after an intensive evaluation via using manner of a healthcare expert focusing on sleep treatment. The suitability of surgical interventions depends at the man or woman's particular anatomical dispositions, severity of sleep apnea, and other factors. Surgical treatments can also have functionality risks and headaches, and their effectiveness can range amongst human beings. Close postoperative observe-up and ongoing monitoring are critical to evaluate remedy effects and address any problems which could get up.

8.2 Types of Sleep Apnea Surgeries

There are severa types of surgeries to be had for the remedy of sleep apnea. The underlying reason specific surgical approach is based upon on the of the sleep apnea and the anatomical

abnormalities contributing to the airway obstruction. Here are a few commonplace varieties of sleep apnea surgical techniques:

Uvulopalatopharyngoplasty (UPPP): UPPP is a surgery that objectives to take away more tissue from the throat, which incorporates the uvula, tonsils, and a part of the soft palate. By reducing the dimensions of those systems, UPPP enables widen the airway and reduce obstructions. It is generally used for humans with obstruction extensively talking inside the mild palate place.

Maxillomandibular Advancement (MMA): MMA is a surgery that repositions the higher and reduce jaws to beautify them ahead. By moving the jaws, the airway vicinity is improved, lowering the collapsibility of the mild tissues within the returned of the throat. MMA is often recommended for individuals with anatomical abnormalities related to the jaw and base of the tongue. Nasal Surgery: Nasal surgical treatment may be executed to correct nasal obstructions that make contributions to sleep apnea. Procedures which include septoplasty (straightening the nasal septum), turbinate cut price (reducing the scale of nasal turbinates), or nasal valve reconstruction can enhance nasal airflow and decrease resistance.

Lingual Tonsillectomy: Lingual tonsillectomy includes doing away with more tissue from the decrease again of the tongue, referred to as the lingual tonsils. This technique is useful for people with large obstruction or increase of the lingual tonsils, that can make a contribution to sleep apnea.

Hyoid Suspension: Hyoid suspension is a surgical procedure that involves repositioning and stabilizing the hyoid bone. The hyoid bone permits the bottom of the tongue and can be a supply of obstruction in some humans. Hyoid suspension permits to boom patency. The balance of the hyoid bone and improve airway

Tracheostomy: Tracheostomy is a surgical treatment wherein a gap is made within the the front of the neck, growing an immediate air passage thru the trachea. It is normally reserved for excessive times of sleep apnea which may be unresponsive to unique remedies. Tracheostomy bypasses the higher airway obstruction genuinely and allows air to go together with the waft proper away into the lungs.

It's critical to observe that the suitability of these surgical processes varies counting on the man or woman's unique situation and underlying anatomical abnormalities. Each surgical operation includes its personal capability risks and advantages. A thorough assessment and consultation with a healthcare expert focusing on sleep medicinal drug are crucial to decide the most suitable surgical technique based totally totally on character needs and treatment desires.

eight.Three Considerations and Success Rates

When considering sleep apnea surgical techniques, it is important to remember various factors and recognize the functionality fulfillment expenses related to those techniques. While surgical interventions can be powerful for some humans, they will not be appropriate or effective for all of us. Here are some issues and a top diploma view of fulfillment expenses associated with sleep apnea surgical strategies:

Severity of Sleep Apnea: The severity of sleep apnea can effect the fulfillment of surgical interventions. Mild to moderate cases can also have better fulfillment costs in comparison to severe cases. It is crucial to go through a complete assessment and talk with a healthcare professional to decide the maximum appropriate remedy approach.

Underlying Anatomy: The anatomical factors contributing to sleep apnea vary amongst people.

Surgical procedures intention particular areas, collectively with the soft palate, tonsils, tongue base, or nasal passages. The achievement of the surgical procedure depends on because it need to be figuring out and addressing the underlying anatomical abnormalities inflicting the obstruction.

Compliance and Adherence: Compliance and adherence to recommended postoperative care and way of existence adjustments are essential for a fulfillment effects. Following postoperative commands, along with preserving a wholesome weight, abstaining from smoking, and adhering to encouraged sleep practices, can make a contribution to the fulfillment of the surgical remedy.

Multidisciplinary Approach: Sleep apnea remedy regularly calls for a multidisciplinary method, related to collaboration among sleep professionals, ENT (Ear, Nose, and Throat) surgeons, and unique healthcare experts. A entire evaluation and custom designed remedy plan are crucial to cope with every body's specific dreams.

Success Rates: Success prices for sleep apnea surgical procedures variety relying on the system completed, the severity and kind of sleep apnea, and character factors. Success is commonly measured thru enhancements in sleep awesome, cut price in the frequency and severity of apneas, and development in symptoms and symptoms. Success fees can range from 40% to 70% for UPPP and 70% to ninety% for MMA, however person stories might also additionally variety.

Combination Therapies: In some cases, aggregate healing procedures may be greater powerful than standalone surgical interventions. Combining surgical procedures with different treatment modalities like first rate airway pressure treatment or oral domestic equipment may additionally additionally moreover decorate treatment results, specifically for human beings with complex sleep apnea or residual signs after surgical operation.

It is critical to talk over with a healthcare professional focusing on sleep medication and an expert health practitioner to discuss the unique issues, potential dangers, advantages, and success charges of sleep apnea surgical procedures. A personalised treatment plan may be advanced based mostly on person needs, severity of sleep apnea, and anatomical factors, deliberating the first-rate to be had evidence and scientific information. Regular comply with-up visits are essential to display development and make any important adjustments to optimize treatment effects.

eight.Four Combination Therapies

Combination treatment plans for sleep apnea contain the simultaneous use of a couple of treatment modalities to deal with the underlying causes and signs and symptoms of the scenario. These techniques reason to optimize remedy consequences and decorate the overall control of sleep apnea. Here's a top degree view of some not unusual aggregate remedies:

Positive Airway Pressure (PAP) Therapy + Therapy: This mixture involves the usage of a strain device, together with non-prevent wonderful Oral Appliance excellent airway airway strain

(CPAP) or bilevel high-quality airway pressure (BiPAP), along element an oral gadget. The PAP remedy allows hold an open airway, whilst the oral equipment helps stabilize the jaw and tongue to prevent airway crumble. This combination can be beneficial for people with every obstructive sleep apnea (OSA) and positional factors or for individuals who discover it difficult to tolerate PAP therapy by myself.

Positive Airway Pressure (PAP) Therapy + Positional Therapy: For individuals with positional obstructive sleep apnea (POSA), combining PAP therapy with positional remedy may be effective. PAP remedy gives continuous wonderful airway pressure to maintain airway patency, at the equal time as positional therapy enables inspire dozing in non-supine positions to lessen positional-associated obstructions.

Positive Airway Pressure (PAP) Therapy + Weight Loss: Weight loss can drastically improve sleep apnea signs and signs and signs, in particular in folks which are obese or obese. Combining PAP therapy with weight reduction interventions, which incorporates nutritional changes and exercise, ought to have additive blessings.

Chapter 9: Choosing The Right Sleep Apnea Device

nine.1 Factors to Consider

When deciding on a snooze apnea device, numerous factors ought to be taken into consideration to make sure the nice healthful for an man or woman's needs and treatment dreams. Here are some vital factors to recollect:

Type of Sleep Apnea: The form of sleep apnea, whether or not or not it's far obstructive sleep apnea (OSA), massive sleep apnea (CSA), or a combination of every, influences the choice of tool. For OSA, first-rate airway pressure (PAP) treatment, oral domestic device, or positional treatment devices can be suitable. For CSA, adaptive servo-air flow (ASV) devices are often encouraged.

Severity of Sleep Apnea: The severity of sleep apnea, as determined with the aid of an character's apnea-hypopnea index (AHI), lets in guide treatment choices. Mild instances can also additionally additionally gain from manner of existence changes or oral home equipment, on the identical time as mild to excessive instances generally require PAP remedy or extra superior devices.

Individual Preferences and Comfort: Individual alternatives play a giant function in device choice. Some humans also can discover PAP remedy mask uncomfortable, who pick possibility alternatives at the side of nasal mask or nasal pillows. Comfort is essential to ensure prolonged-term adherence and effective treatment consequences.

Mask Fit and Size: For PAP remedy, deciding on the right masks in shape and length is important. The mask should form a solid seal without causing soreness or air leaks. Different mask patterns, consisting of complete face, nasal, or nasal pillow masks, offer numerous ranges of coverage and can be decided on primarily based totally on non-public desire and facial shape.

Lifestyle and Mobility: Considerations regarding way of life and mobility want to be considered. Individuals who regularly journey or have an lively way of life also can furthermore choose out portable or travelfriendly devices. Additionally, noise stages and ease of use have to be evaluated whilst deciding on a tool.

Insurance Coverage and Cost: Understanding coverage insurance and related prices is crucial. Different devices have numerous costs, and insurance coverage may also additionally furthermore vary relying on the unique device and character insurance plans. Considering budget constraints and walking with coverage organizations can help find out the maximum reasonably-priced alternatives.

Healthcare Provider Recommendations: Seeking steerage from healthcare vendors, which include sleep professionals or durable medical tool providers, is critical.

They can verify individual desires, offer tool tips, and assist in finding the most suitable device for effective treatment.

It is important to have a examine that device choice may additionally additionally require a tribulation-anderror manner, as person responses can range. Regular take a look at-up visits with healthcare agencies are critical to assess treatment efficacy, deal with any issues, and make important modifications to optimize remedy effects.

9.2 Consultation with Healthcare Professionals

Consultation with healthcare professionals is a crucial step in dealing with sleep apnea effectively. Healthcare professionals focusing on sleep medicine, including sleep professionals or sleep medication physicians, play a significant role in the analysis, treatment, and ongoing control of sleep apnea. Here's an define of the significance of session with healthcare specialists:

Accurate Diagnosis: Sleep apnea could have severa underlying motives and contributing factors.

Consulting with a healthcare professional lets in ensure an accurate evaluation with the resource of conducting a entire assessment, which can also include an in depth medical records, physical examination, and sleep observe. Proper assessment is important to increase the proper remedy plan.

Treatment Guidance: Healthcare experts offer expert guidance on remedy options based on an character's specific sleep apnea diagnosis, severity, and special elements. They can speak the professionals and cons of severa remedy modalities, educate human beings about available alternatives, and assist make informed alternatives.

Customized Treatment Plans: Sleep apnea manage requires custom designed treatment plans tailor-made to person goals. Healthcare specialists take into account factors which encompass the sort and severity of sleep apnea, the presence of comorbidities, way of lifestyles elements, and private options while designing remedy plans. They take a holistic method to deal with all elements of sleep apnea manipulate.

Treatment Monitoring and Adjustments: Healthcare specialists show remedy progress and make vital changes to optimize treatment outcomes.

They compare treatment efficacy via observe-up visits, display compliance with treatment, decide treatment-associated element consequences, and make appropriate changes to remedy modalities or tool settings as wished.

Education and Support: Healthcare professionals provide schooling and help to human beings with sleep apnea. They offer an reason for the importance of treatment adherence, provide data on way of life modifications, sleep hygiene practices, and answer any questions or issues. They act as a precious useful aid at some point of the treatment adventure, imparting steerage and encouragement.

Collaboration with Other Specialists: Sleep apnea may be related to different scientific situations, which encompass cardiovascular disease, weight issues, or diabetes. Healthcare professionals collaborate with specific professionals, collectively with cardiologists, pulmonologists, or dentists, to manipulate the ones comorbidities and ensure complete care.

Consulting with healthcare professionals guarantees that people get hold of evidence-based care, customized remedy plans, and ongoing guide for their sleep apnea manage. Regular study-up visits and open communique with healthcare corporations are crucial to monitor improvement, deal with any concerns or challenges, and optimize remedy outcomes for progressed sleep great and ordinary properly-being.

9.Three Insurance Coverage and Costs

Insurance coverage and costs are critical issues while

trying to find treatment for sleep apnea. Understanding your coverage coverage and the associated expenses will permit you to navigate the monetary elements of sleep apnea control effectively. Here's an outline of coverage coverage and expenses related to sleep apnea:

Insurance Coverage: Many insurance plans provide coverage for the analysis and treatment of sleep apnea. This coverage may moreover encompass diagnostic sleep research, visits to sleep specialists, and various treatment options which includes top notch airway stress (PAP) treatment, oral home gadget, and surgical interventions. The scope of insurance, but, may additionally moreover vary based totally at the insurance organization and the precise plan.

Chapter 10: How Sleep Builds Our Brains And Bodies

In this monetary ruin, you'll find out:

A short assessment of sleep levels

A brief summary of the advantages of sleep.

If you'd like to dig deeper, try my e-book, Airway is Life, or look at Why We Sleep with the useful resource of Matthew Walker, Ph.D.

I changed into starting to get a piece depressed approximately my patients' health. I observed the identical human beings three hundred and sixty five days after twelve months, and it simply regarded like they have been in decline. Even patients my age without a doubt saved including new health troubles to the listing. Their tooth and gums have been affected, of direction, but it have emerge as pretty obvious that dental problems had been a symptom of the ailment gadget, not the cause.

Sometimes, sleep seems almost like a punishment. You're a busy person with activities! You have new matters to research, chores to capture up on, youngsters to take care of, a exercise you need to expand, and what approximately amusing? Shouldn't you've got were given some time to lighten up? Instead, each and every night time, you need to forestall the whole thing you're doing and go to sleep, in any other case you'll pay for it later.

It's no wonder toddlers fight sleep. Sleep is stopping. Sleep is stupid. Sleep isn't always a few thing, only a pause, right? Wrong. Sleep is what keeps us healthful, glad and human. We need sleep to function at our fantastic. When college university university students pull all-nighters or busy mothers live up late binge-searching Netflix, they may suppose that they're the usage of their time correctly.

In reality, they're crippling their thoughts and body. You need sleep nearly as loads as you need food. Good sleep restores you, solidifies new learning, and protects your body from damage. There's a reason the Geneva

Convention lists sleep deprivation as a form of torture.

To put in force sleep treatment for your dental exercise, you're going to want a exquisite statistics of what sleep is and the manner healthy sleep makes healthful humans. If you've already attended my direction or look at my ebook Airway is Life, an entire lot of this could be evaluation for you. Otherwise, get prepared for a whirlwind tour thru Sleep one zero one.

What Sleep Looks Like to A Scientist

Sleep technological know-how is a reasonably new field. We didn't truly have the tools to study sleep till the mid-20th century. By 1957, we'd discovered that there are 5 degrees of sleep, divided into NREM and REM. The thoughts movements via those styles of stages throughout the night time time, and our frame dreams all 5 stages to live healthful.

Stage zero: When You're Awake

When you are large unsleeping, your thoughts waves, coronary coronary heart fee, respiratory, and frame temperature are continuously in flux. You're searching round, responding to the arena, dashing up and slowing down, and constantly changing. You're taking in and processing records, ingesting and processing meals, and shifting spherical constantly. The great regular is exchange.

NREM Stage 1: Drifting Off

After an extended day, you in the end have a risk to lie down. You sink into your pillow and close to your eyes. Within a few minutes, your respiration and coronary coronary heart rate gradual. Your frame temperature starts to drop. Your brainwaves alternate too. They grow to be decrease voltage than your daylight hours symptoms, and their pattern starts offevolved to change.

In Stage 1, your thoughts end up more random and pressured. You save you records the conversations and sounds spherical you. If a person wakes you up, you may now not undergo in mind having slept in any respect. In level one, you may revel in "sleep jerks," wherein you experience like you are falling or thrashing and jerk yourself extensive awake.

Most people spend amongst 1 and 7 mins on this stage of mild sleep. For instance, at the same time as an exhausted new determine takes catnaps wherein they waft off for a couple of minutes within the middle of hard work or chores, they are hitting this stage of sleep. After you have got spent severa minutes in Stage 1 NREM, your brainwaves exchange all over again, and you've got entered Stage 2.

Stage 2 NREM: Light Sleep

In Stage 2 NREM, your brainwaves begin forming "sleep spindles." If someone wakes you sooner or later of Stage 2, you've got top notch been in a mild sleep. You can wake up and revel in refreshed however the reality that you have not completed a whole sleep cycle. Many '"energy naps'" take benefit of a quick period of Stage 2 sleep.

You'll stay on this degree for ten to 20-5 mins. Slowly, the sleep spindles becomes fewer, and the thoughts waves take on the slow, rhythmic patterns that suggest which you've slipped right right into a deeper sleep.

Stages 3 and 4 NREM: Deep Sleep

Some scientists distinguish amongst Stage three and Stage four NREM, while others say that they may be every components of the same deep sleep. During those degrees, a wholesome character studies sluggish, ordinary respiratory, a slow coronary coronary heart rate, and synchronized, slow delta brain waves. This is the sleep you need to sense sincerely and without a doubt rested.

If you are a parent, you have got were given probably visible a little one or child in a deep sleep. This is when they pass limp. You can elevate their arm, and it truely falls lower back into vicinity. You can flow into them spherical from a automobile to a bed, and they by no means even stir. Deeply sound asleep adults may be tough to wake too, however their brains are however open to environmental stimuli. Researchers have determined that during quick intervals inside the direction of every thoughts wave, the brain can respond to outdoor noises. So, even while you're deeply asleep, you may even though hear the weird crash outside, the crying toddler, or the smoke alarm. Your mind is designed to keep you safe, even whilst you're sleeping.

This degree commonly lasts from 20-forty minutes. It ends with a move back to Stage 2 for five-10 mins. After revisiting Stage 2, you don't cross lower lower back to Stage 1. Instead, you enter a nation called REM.

REM: The Dreaming State

In REM, or speedy eye motion sleep, your mind is as energetic as while you're enormous wakeful. Sometimes it is even extra energetic. Your eyes flow hastily, however the rest of your frame memories a form of paralysis, so you may not flow spherical and damage your self on the identical time as you are dreaming. The rational facilities of your mind are suppressed, but your emotional centers are strolling the show. The quantity of time you spend in REM is based upon on the sleep cycle you are in. At the begin of the night time time, your periods of REM are very quick. Then, due to the fact the night time time is going on and you entire more sleep cycles, you spend an increasing number of time in REM.

Sleep Cycles

Your mind moves among Stage 2, deep sleep, and REM sleep all night time time extended. Over the course of a superb night time's sleep, you'll spend about half the time in Stage 2. In every ninety-minute duration, you can enjoy Stage 2, Stages three and four, and REM sleep. About 4 hours into your sleep, you can awaken and in quick pass round, use the rest room, or get a drink of water. Then you'll start lower again at Stage 1 and begin once more.

Hypnograms

A hypnogram is a diagram displaying whilst a sleeper is in every degree and the way lengthy they spend there. Sleep experts can have a have a look at hypnograms to find out problems in a person's sleep. For example, a loss of deep sleep or an excessive amount of REM too early within the night time can help diagnose a sleep problem.

Hypnograms also are useful for coaching your group and patients approximately healthy sleep and the way our thoughts actions amongst stages of sleep.

I had a extremely good rapport with my sufferers, and I favored to assist them. They had been all seeing a couple of experts who never talked to each distinct. Their fitness issues had been being handled in isolation; however there has been a few issue large occurring. I in reality wasn't certain what I, as a dentist, should do to help, and it turn out to be traumatic.

What Healthy Sleep Does for the Brain, Body, and Moods?

Why are scientists so interested in sleep? Because the more we have a look at it, the extra vital it gets. We're continuously finding out approximately new methods that sleep protects our our our bodies and our brains. For instance, many researchers who take a look at autism spectrum issues know that, at the foundation, a few children with ASD might also moreover furthermore have underlying sleep troubles that purpose or exacerbate their signs and signs and symptoms. We're finding sleep hyperlinks with highbrow ailments as well. And many bodily troubles may have their roots in awful sleep. It's impossible to offer a whole listing of the whole thing sleep does to your mind and body. What follows is a short listing to jog your reminiscence and assist you teach your organization and sufferers.

Chapter 11: Sleep Regulates Hormones

Bodies aren't built to be "on" 24-7. They want a length of sleep each day to reset, restore, and renew. Some of the hormones sleep regulates consist of:

Human Growth Hormone - HGH is released in the route of gradual-wave sleep early in the night time time. In youngsters, it lets in them develop larger. In adults, it causes the frame to restore and replace damaged cells, it breaks down fat for electricity, and it helps the frame collect muscle. When someone is trying to shed pounds however staying up overdue, they're reducing the effectiveness of HGH and making their dreams extra hard to gather.

Cortisol - Cortisol is the stress hormone. The body suppresses it in a few unspecified time inside the destiny of sleep so that all of the frame's structures get a smash from 'combat or flight.'

Ghrelin - Ghrelin is the hormone that makes people sense hungry. When a person sleeps well, it's suppressed. Good sleep way no midnight snack cravings.

Leptin - Leptin is the hormone that promotes feelings of satiety. It's improved at some point of sleep in order that the sleeper feels complete and burns power.

The following chart sums up the hormonal movement of sleep. Keep it available for speaking for your patients and crew individuals!

Sleep and Learning

Sleep is crucial for mastering. During the day, all the senses take in data, we bear in mind it, and we try to analyze new things. Sleep is whilst the mind consolidates our learning truly so we will use it later. There are some precise strategies wherein sleep lets in us test:

Clearing out the fast-term reminiscence - Our short-time period reminiscence is primarily based definitely inside the hypothalamus. This part of the thoughts high-quality has a constrained amount of garage region, like a photo card in a digital digital camera. When it receives complete, we truely can't studies anymore. This is why small youngsters need naps. Everything is new to them, so their hypothalamus runs out of location quick. This is also why students analyzing for a large test will enjoy like their brain is actually whole. They need a burst of NREM sleep to keep mastering. This approach can happen pretty quick, it absolutely is why a energy nap can regularly wake up an beaten thoughts.

Storing new know-how where it can be retrieved - Slow-wave sleep types and shops new information simply so the mind can retrieve it even as you want it. Without sleep, you could research new matters, however they may not be clean to keep in mind. This is why pulling all-nighters earlier than exams is counterproductive for university kids.

Practicing new motor skills - Muscle memory is truly motor planning reminiscence. Your mind has to learn how to ship a chain of commands to your muscle groups to complete a task. Sleep is wherein your thoughts practices these sequences of actions so that you can art work perfectly while awake. Because the frame is paralyzed in the course of deep sleep, this motor practice does now not result in real actions.

Refining memories and forgetting unimportant facts - A few days after you have got a look at some element new, your mind will refine the memory, preserving and strengthening the important additives at the same time as forgetting extraneous records.

Repairing and rewiring the mind - Neuroplasticity is a result of the artwork that takes area inside the direction of sleep. This rewiring, repairing, and interconnection occurs during REM sleep.

Learning to navigate social situations and complicated emotions - REM sleep is how the thoughts learns to navigate social and emotional problems. Since extra REM occurs at the cease of your night time time of sleep, those who habitually awaken to early are lacking out on essential social and emotional gaining knowledge of.

Creative trouble-solving - Your thoughts works on troubles on the same time as you sleep, this is why humans regularly provide you with a high-quality solution first element in the morning. As the mind types information and makes new connections, it creates solutions that you virtually could not have been capable of take into account the night time before.

This is just a short precis of some of the greater crucial matters that sleep does for our bodies and our brains. Since sleep is such an important part of our lives, shouldn't we want all of our patients, and absolutely all people we adore, to be getting their quality viable sleep every night time time of their lives?

When I took Dr. Dassani's magnificence, the quantities started out out to fall into place. There changed into an underlying motive for the ones signs and symptoms and signs, and I, as a dentist, must assist them in tactics that their specialists couldn't. Sleep Medicine have emerge as the missing link inside the chain of experts, and I may want to assist them in my workplace, with the environment and group they already knew and cherished.

Implementation on Target!

After this bankruptcy, you'll need to do the subsequent to get on direction in your sleep dentistry exercise:

Learn the levels of sleep, and what they do for the frame, with the useful resource of coronary coronary heart. You have to be capable of provide an explanation for the ones in your company and patients with out notes. Knowing your fabric makes you extra persuasive.

Learn the hormone adjustments with sleep.

Be capable of offer an cause of to dad and mom, in reality and concisely, why loss of sleep impacts their kids's sports sports and teachers.

If you're a script individual, now's the time to start writing your scripts. However, I favor to apprehend the material interior and out, in order that the affected individual and I may additionally have a communique, not a lecture.

Sleep Breathing: Structural Issues in Children and Adults

In this monetary disaster you can locate:

Descriptions of OSA and UARS

Explanations of methods the tonsils and adenoids obstruct the pediatric airway

Why tongue tie and immoderate palates are essential

How the mild palate contributes to OSA in adults

How the tongue and jaw have an effect on the person airway

Why neck length topics

My husband had snored for years, in all likelihood as long as we'd been married. I didn't assume a notable deal of it, because of the reality he'd generally been that manner and I ought to poke him even as he had to roll over. The first-rate trouble became that he have been given common sinus infections, and at the same time as the ones hit there has been not something anyone should do for his respiratory. They took a huge toll, however his ENT had no answers other than 'extra steroids.' So we lived with it.

There are many motives of disrupted sleep, which includes:

Circadian Rhythm troubles

Clock genes

Lack of the hormone melatonin

Poor sleep hygiene

Difficult work schedules

Mental contamination

Acid Reflux

In our practices, our predominant cognizance need to be figuring out people losing sleep because of obstructive sleep apnea (OSA). OSA happens while structural troubles restrict the airway. Because the airway is in part or in truth blocked, the frame can't get sufficient oxygen. The sleeper struggles to respire, wakes up for a few seconds, and then slips yet again into sleep. These microarousals are so brief that the sleeper will no longer take into account them within the morning. However, the paintings of sleep is disrupted.

We need to moreover discover sufferers with pinnacle airway resistance syndrome (UARS). UARS is usually a precursor to OSA, wherein the affected individual struggles to transport air via the pinnacle airways, however can nevertheless get enough airflow to hold oxygen levels. However, UARS patients want to art work greater difficult to respire and the war effects in microarousals or longer waking durations in the course of the night time.

Because sleep is disrupted, the frame starts offevolved a downward spiral that, if untreated, will in the long run result in OSA. By figuring out and treating sufferers with UARS, we are able to halt the infection approach and help them keep away from the burden advantage, metabolic, and cardiovascular troubles due to OSA.

If we will perceive the structural issues inflicting terrible sleep, we are capable of accurate them. Dentists are the precise companies to select out and deal with OSA because of the truth we art work with jaws, palates, tooth, and tongues. In maximum instances of OSA, those are the elements of the frame which may be causing or contributing to the obstruction. If a affected person to your administrative center fails a snooze display, you'll need to conduct a bodily exam to understand the source of the problems.

Chapter 12: Common Obstructions In Pediatric Patients

For youngsters with OSA, the tonsils, adenoids, tongue, and palate are frequently the culprits.

Tonsils and Adenoids

Tonsils and Adenoids are frequently notably enlarged in pediatric patients with OSA or UARS. These obstruct the airway, in particular even as the kid is drowsing on their back. They are the sort of commonplace cause of obstruction that the number one line of treatment for a kid with OSA is often to eliminate them. However, mouth-respiratory also can purpose the tonsils and adenoids to swell, so it's crucial to ensure that there isn't a greater primary purpose to the respiration issues.

Tongue

The tongue is supposed to relaxation at the roof of the mouth inside the path of sleep. If it does no longer, it is able to fall backward and obstruct the stroke. In cutting-edge-day years, increasingly kids were offering with OSA due to an unrevised tongue-tie (ankyloglossia). This is because pediatricians and midwives have stopped revising ties till there may be a smooth problem with boom and feeding. However, even youngsters who don't have feeding troubles in infancy can later have sleep issues because of tongue-tie and horrible tongue positioning.

Palate

A immoderate, slender tough palate can prevent respiration by means of using using decreasing the volume of the nasal hollow space. With the reduced extent, a slight cold or allergic reactions may be enough to dam off airflow and reason mouth-respiratory and frequent night-waking. Often, a infant with an unrevised tongue-tie can even have palate problems, as a ordinary tongue acts as a palate expander within the early years.

Common Causes of Obstruction in Adult Patients with OSA

In adults with OSA, the maximum not unusual reasons of obstruction are the clean palate, the tongue, the jaw, and the tissue surrounding the neck.

Soft Palate

As human beings age, they virtually lose muscle tone of their mild palates. During sleep, a floppy palate can completely or in component ward off the pinnacle airway, main to mouth breathing or sleep apneas.

The Tongue

There are three primary techniques in which the tongue can have an effect on an adult airway at some point of sleep:

Unrevised tongue tie - We're starting to see an increasing number of adults whose tongue ties had been no longer revised as infants. This can result in the same troubles with sleep respiratory that it does in a infant due to the fact the tongue can't rest on the palate within the course of sleep. Even in adults, revising a tongue tie (determined with the aid of myofunctional remedy to investigate new abilties), can decorate sleep respiration.

Fatty tongue - When human beings benefit weight, they gain it everywhere, which incorporates on their tongues. A 2020 take a look at from the University of Pennsylvania positioned that dropping fat at the tongue significantly advanced sleep apnea.

Bad behavior - If a person has fallen into the dependancy of mouth-respiratory (probably from persistent sinus or allergic reaction problems) they will have moreover misplaced the addiction of proper tongue positioning all through sleep. Some studies endorse that tongue bodily video video games can alleviate this trouble and improve sleep apnea.

Retrognathia

A recessed jaw impacts sleep respiratory as it forces the tongue yet again into the throat eventually of sleep. This narrows or blocks the airway, and can reason apneas. For sufferers with mild retrognathia, there are oral home equipment available to put the jaw for extra steady sleep.

Neck Size

When there are fatty deposits within the neck, they could compress the airway in a few unspecified time within the destiny of sleep and purpose apneas. Adult girls whose necks are extra than sixteen inches round and person men whose necks are more than 17 inches round are at excessive danger for OSA.

Both of our kids had had tongue ties. I'd revised them myself, and they'd moreover every wanted maxillary growth. I knew my husband had had tooth pulled even as he have been given braces as a child. I knew our children breathed a bargain better after I'd steady their palates, however I'd in no way related the dots. I turned into too stuck in considering tongue-tie and palate issues as a pediatric problem. After the elegance, I observed out that now not pleasant did a number of my sufferers want treatment for sleep respiration problems, however that my husband did too. The class saved his life and his fitness.

Why Doesn't Everyone with Obstructions Have Full-blown OSA?

Sometimes a affected individual has bodily capabilities which can contribute to sleep apnea however can pass a sleep check in a lab. This is due to the fact OSA frequently requires multiple failures at distinct elements in the higher respiration syndrome. So a affected character may moreover have UARS and battle to respire, however not have whole-blow OSA.

On the alternative hand, any other exchange such as weight advantage, excessive hypersensitivity problems, or possibly an damage can then be sufficient to tip someone over into sleep apnea. It's crucial to end up aware about treatable bodily issues early in order that OSA and its headaches may be averted.

Implementation on Target!

After this economic disaster, you should start considering how you can encompass sleep-disordered respiration (SDB) displays into your person and pediatric tests. For instance:

Will you show display all new pediatric sufferers for tongue-tie?

Will you alert parents to palate troubles?

Will you check the tonsils and tongue?

For adults, will you diploma neck period?

How will you cope with evidence of an overbite?

What is probably your reaction to signs and symptoms of enamel-grinding?

Think approximately these elements of the manner OSA offers and start planning how your assessments will change. Later, it'll probable be essential so you can estimate how a awesome deal time sleep dentistry opinions will upload to new patient and returning affected individual appointments.

three: Sleep Breathing: How Bad Sleep Affects Children

In this financial disaster, you can examine:

Why sleep problems can appearance so high-quality in precise children

Common signs and signs and symptoms of pediatric SDB

Why mouth-respiratory is an especially big hassle

My exercise had such a whole lot of kids getting identified with ADHD, ODD, and precise conduct problems. But looking on the dad and mom, they didn't have a data with those troubles. It's like the kids' hassle just got here from nowhere. It struck me as abnormal. With some kids who've the ones diagnoses, you take a look at the child, after which the dad and mom and siblings, and you can see how that is a circle of relatives trait. But with some? It appeared instantly, and I questioned if some element else become happening.

Do you have got were given any kids for your workout who've sleep-disordered respiration (SDB)? If you observe pediatric sufferers, you almost actually do. SDB impacts approximately three% of children beneath 12 inside the US, however maximum kids are hardly ever screened for it.

One reason that dad and mom and caregivers don't have children evaluated for sleep breathing issues is that a sleepless infant does not normally act like a sleepless man or woman. For example, study those "day in a lifestyles" memories for 2 unique youngsters.

Linnea the Lazy

Linnea have become an lively toddler, however as a seven-year-vintage, she's without a doubt lazy. She whines approximately chores. She whines approximately walks. She whines about getting up in the morning. She has a terrible urge for meals and pleasant wants to devour easy carbs like crackers, chips, and fruit snacks. At home, she's constantly bored till she's allowed to have a look at her desired indicates. She slumps on the sofa together along with her mouth open, gazing monitors.

At university, Linnea spends an entire lot of time at the side of her head on her desk. She's gradual to speak, sluggish to examine, and slow to do math. She can't observe -step commands and regularly loses her vicinity. Whenever she's requested a query, her reply is "I don't don't forget." Sometimes, she breaks down crying for no precise cause. Her circle of relatives is first-rate, and her siblings are normal kids. No you'll discern out what's wrong with Linnea. "Well," her instructor says, "I bet there's one in each circle of relatives."

Rex the Rowdy

Rex is a ball of normal strength and horrific life alternatives. If there's a pool, he's the only screaming "Cannonball!" and leaping in and ruining everybody's swim. If there's a dare, he'll take it. He's in the ER so frequently his mother has joked they have to call a bay after him. Rex runs through life at entire tempo, by no means slowing down, no matter the truth that he runs into something. His mom attempted to region him in sports sports to expend some of the electricity, however Rex couldn't have a look at commands, indignant his teammates, and had maximum vital meltdowns whenever he changed into thwarted.

At university, Rex is the child with the table within the nook so he received't disrupt the work of the alternative students. He shouts out answers as fast as a query is asked, and is usually wrong. He in no manner completes art work, he received't sit although, and he's constantly acting out and getting out of his seat. His teacher desires she need to suggest an ADHD evaluation at the following decide-teacher conference because of the reality she without a doubt can't take his behavior anymore.

Which this sort of children has OSA? The solution may be "Both of them!" When a little one is out of sync and now not getting right sleep, one of a kind variables much like the circle of relatives manner of existence, the child's man or woman, and comorbid conditions all play a feature in how they behave and what problems they have got.

Chapter 13: Spotting Sdb In Kids

After the seminar, I observed the pattern. These kids had been kids who weren't drowsing, and who had super troubles with respiratory. The first dad and mom I approached about sleep remedy had been those who had those kids due to the fact I desired to help the kids who were struggling maximum first.

Red flags for a sleep-disadvantaged little one consist of:

A routine mouth breather - Children breathe thru their mouths on the equal time as their noses and sinuses are obstructed.

Slack-jawed posture - When a infant is slack-jawed it can signify bad oral muscle control or horrible conduct, and each of these can intrude with sleep respiration.

Whiny with low electricity stages - This is an indication of a infant who isn't getting enough sleep or who isn't respiratory nicely enough to have electricity.

Dampened emotions, bored with the whole thing -

An exhausted toddler is simply too worn-out to be happy, interested, or even irritated.

Bed-wetting - Frequent microarousals purpose the bladder to lose control. Often the hassle with bedwetters isn't that they sleep too deeply, however they by no means sleep deeply sufficient to pay interest urine in their sleep.

Poor college simple overall performance - If a little one isn't slumbering, it may be difficult for them to grasp new material or undergo in mind familiar fabric quick.

Hyperactivity - Some sleep-disadvantaged kids are hyperactive. They are in search of everyday stimulus to stay wide awake and alert, much like an person could in all likelihood shake themselves, soar up and down, or splash bloodless water on their face. However, for the reason that youngsters are immature this stimulation takes the form of strolling, bouncing, speaking, and performing out inappropriately.

Poor emotional control, collectively with meltdowns - Emotional control takes recognition, specially for greater youthful youngsters. A sleep-deprived toddler is on an emotional rollercoaster.

Difficulty navigating peer relationships - A sleep-disadvantaged baby isn't learning the abilities to interact with pals and isn't able to nicely method social interactions.

Clumsiness and poor potential to investigate new gross motor skills - Motor studying requires appropriate sufficient sleep. A sleep-disadvantaged baby will frequently lag at the back of pals in gross motor capabilities.

Restless sleep with hundreds of tossing and turning - Kids with sleep problems regularly glide loads in their sleep, get twisted of their sheets, and fling their our bodies spherical all night time.

Sensory searching out or sensory avoidant behaviors - Some youngsters react to exhaustion with the aid of the use of searching out strain, spinning, or looking for thrilling textures and sounds. Others near down and contact for silence, familiarity, and dim rooms. However, in both instances, the conduct is rooted in not being capable of awareness or manipulate their emotions.

Snoring - While loud night breathing isn't commonly a sign of disordered breathing in a infant, it can be an vital indicator.

Dark circles under the eyes - We additionally call those "hypersensitive reaction eyes" or "raccoon eyes." When a infant has those dark circles, it way some factor is interrupting their sleep.

Anxiety - Sleepless youngsters are annoying. They recognise they may be lacking subjects, forgetting subjects, and being asked to do things they may be capable of't do, and that they don't recognize WHY they may't act like one of a kind kids.

Space cadet - Focus and quick-time period reminiscence undergo whilst a toddler doesn't sleep. So they get tagged as a vicinity cadet who can't preserve subjects in their mind. They lose their location in obligations effects, and may't keep in thoughts what comes next.

Morning headaches - Kids with breathing issues often wake dry-mouthed and with a headache.

Always catching breathing bugs - Kids with sleep respiration troubles frequently breathe thru their mouths at night time. Without the nostril to humidify, smooth, and heat the air, they're sending too-dry, too bloodless, germ-laden air into their lungs. They worsen their throat and lungs and depart themselves more vulnerable to coughs and colds.

When a determine comes into your workplace, and also you every see a number of the ones symptoms and symptoms and symptoms in a toddler or they're indexed at the assessment, it's time to talk to the own family approximately sleep-disordered breathing. Often the ones mother and father have had no idea what is inaccurate with their infant, or that there might be a not unusual thread connecting them. Sometimes the terrible little one has been subjected to infinite vicinity in an try to trade behaviors that they've no manipulate over. When you perceive a infant with sleep-disordered respiration, you convert lives.

Is Mouth-Breathing Really That Bad?

"Mouth-breather" is an insult flung in political arguments, but why is it so horrible at the equal time as a child can't use her nostril to respire? They're however breathing, right? To understand in reality how destructive mouth-respiration may be to a infant's development, it enables to look at the manner it develops, why it maintains, and what it does to the airlines, and in the end, to mind and body fitness.

How Mouth Breathing Starts

Mouth breathing normally begins offevolved offevolved while the nose and sinus cavities are blocked. The infant can't get air thru their nostril, really so they shift to their mouth. When the problem is a plague, mouth respiratory is normally brief-lived, and parents can take steps like steaming bathrooms or drugs to open up the nostril. When the mouth-breathing is the quit end result of a longer-term hassle like excessive hypersensitive reactions or a immoderate, slim palate that obstructs the nasal hollow region, large problems stop result.

What Happens Next

If the mouth-breathing results from a persistent state of affairs, the kid will form a addiction of mouth respiration. This motives several different troubles with the airway.

The nose and sinuses are crucial for warming and humidifying the air which you breathe. The nose moreover removes particles like dust, mildew, pollen, bacteria, and viruses from the air. And, of course, it permits us to fragrance and enhances our feel of flavor.

When a toddler breathes via her mouth, the air enters the airway "untreated." The air irritates the tonsils, adenoids, and throat, inflicting contamination, swelling, and pain. It enters the decrease airway untreated and effects in extra inflammation and infection.

Mouth-respiration kids are extra at danger for bronchitis, reactive airlines, and bronchial bronchial asthma due to the reality their noses can't do their method. They're moreover extra at chance for enlarged tonsils and adenoids.

Mouth respiration positions the tongue low inside the mouth in location of at the roof of the mouth. This prevents the palate from growing nicely as the kid grows and additionally reasons the tongue to block the airway for the duration of sleep, interfering with sleep respiratory.

Mouth respiratory makes making a music and speaking more tough. Try it. You grow to be gasping for breath over and over.

Mouth breathing can reason a toddler to swallow air, and bring about GI ache.

Mouth breathing even interferes with eating and vitamins. Kids who breathe via their mouths are often chokers. They have hassle chewing and swallowing food and drink due to the fact they could't consume and breathe at the same time. Plus, with out the nostril, food is sincerely much much less palatable. These youngsters will crave amazing-candy and terrific-salty food because of the fact that's what they are able to flavor.

It all offers as a whole lot as a infant who can't breathe, sleep, or eat well. And so these kids get sick more, they're generally worn-out, they warfare with conduct and schoolwork. The longer the mouth-respiratory keeps, the more they pass over out on and the farther they fall within the lower back of. And whilst mouth breathing is a dependancy, it takes effort and time to begin nostril-respiratory once more, even after any underlying problems are corrected. When you spot a mouth-breather for your exercising, it's a sign that they want your assist.

The first affected person we handled have become a revelation. She had an unrevised tongue tie and wanted her palate progressed, and the consequences were extremely good. As she moved away from mouthbreathing and her nasal hole space elevated, her individual modified. Her parents were amazed because of the reality, internal this rage-stuffed, oppositional infant, a candy-tempered little female have grow to be struggling to respire and to relaxation. Now, I ensure to emphasize to mother and father – "Kids who don't act properly possibly don't sense well."

Implementation on Target!

After this bankruptcy, do the following to help you get organized for implementation:

Start developing or collecting educational substances for the mother and father of your sufferers. You'll want diagrams and hand-outs to provide an purpose of why their little one's signs and symptoms and signs and symptoms are complicated. Virtual or physical 3-d models are specifically helpful for explaining the placement of the palate and tongue in respiration.

Start screening for mouth respiration. One quick question to mother and father, or virtually searching the kid breathe, can clue you and your group into larger issues.

Ask approximately faculty, behavioral troubles, and parent troubles. Many dad and mom go into the dentist questioning "this is about tooth," so in case you ask, "do you have got were given were given any questions or problems," they'll simplest reply based at the enamel. Change the manner you speak to mother and father so that you can draw out critical records.

Chapter 14: Sleep Breathing How Bad Sleep

Affects Adults

If you find out sleep-disordered inhaling a toddler, they're probable to get treated brief. Parents need their kids to feel better and achieve success. Adults, alternatively, will often permit UARS or OSA go untreated for a long time. They're busy, the case isn't pressing, sleep research are difficult, they'll get spherical to it later.

When you're coping with character sufferers, it's essential that they understand that untreated sleep breathing troubles are very volatile. It's no longer truely lengthy-time period troubles like diabetes or cardiovascular ailment. Sleep apnea is carefully related to lethal car accidents. Not slumbering puts you prone to falling asleep at the wheel.

My workout had gotten busy. My existence had gotten busy. I'd come home from the exercise, run children to sports activities and help with homework, and collapse into bed. I actually have grow to be jogging so hard to be an engaged company for my sufferers, a glad supervisor for my team, and a top notch mother to my children. Of course, I modified into exhausted and run down and strolling on espresso. That modified into normal, proper?

OSA and UARS are less hard to diagnose in adults than in children, clearly because of the truth the symptoms commonly usually tend to differ less in adults.

Mike's Story

Mike end up in his 50s at the identical time as he came to our exercise. He'd acquired weight in center age and had truly been diagnosed with excessive blood pressure and pre-diabetes. He turn out to be worried due to the truth he'd been grinding his tooth, and because of the fact his associate complained about, "snores that shook the window panes." Mike worked in a production facility, and these days he'd been falling asleep on his strength domestic from art work and spacing out within the route of the day. Mike expected to move away with a mouth protect for tooth-grinding, but as an alternative, we despatched him to a snooze lab. He had a easy case of OSA. Getting remedy proper away advanced his daytime sleepiness, and inner a few months he have become no longer pre-diabetic and his blood stress modified into below control.

Gina's Story

Gina emerge as worn-out all the time, but she become moreover a completely busy individual. She worked out, she had an energetic task, and she had small kids at home. She became narrow and trim, however she actually felt unhealthy. Every time she got a cold, it lingered, from time to time for weeks. She slept 8 hours every night time time time, however she tossed and grew to end up and her husband complained that she snored a bit, occasionally. She had dark circles beneath her eyes that makeup couldn't cover. But on the identical time as she talked to her medical physician about her problems, he couldn't find any evidence of an underlying hassle. "It's honestly some time of life," he defined. "You're busy, you've have been given small children, you're over 30 now. This is truely what takes region." By the time Gina came to us about TMJ issues, she'd given up on getting her power again. Maybe she without a doubt changed into slower and lots less active than her friends and could need to discover ways to stay with it.

OSA is Easy, UARS is Often Overlooked

Mike is a textbook OSA case. He'll have no hassle getting treatment as speedy as he receives screened and also you convince him that he needs assist. Gina is a more difficult case. She's laid low with UARS, no longer complete-blown OSA. This approach that she's suffering to breathe at night, but she still receives sufficient oxygen constantly. The trouble is that for a person with UARS, the conflict to hold respiration triggers microarousals and they toss, turn, and change role. Remember, to do the art work of sleep, the body wants to STAY asleep. Gina's microarousals advise that her body and mind can't heal the way they should. Her hormones are out of whack due to the reality she's no longer dozing deeply enough for prolonged sufficient. Right now, she is healthful, but if she can't get help the damage will pile up. She'll turn out to be with cardiovascular sickness, T2 Diabetes, weight problems, and full-blown OSA due to the reality she isn't always slumbering.

In some approaches, a UARS affected character will achieve a GREATER advantage from treatment than an OSA affected man or woman will due to the fact if you may capture sleep respiration troubles early, you may prevent persistent ailments like diabetes.

So, the sleep route changed into eye-beginning. I identified myself in the signs and symptoms and found out that I'd been assuming OSA modified into for vintage, slow, obese humans, now not younger, trim, energetic moms of their 30s! I changed into my non-public first sleep patient due to the fact I wanted my energy back. I wasn't one hundred% provided on making sleep dentistry a first-rate cognizance of my practice, however I started out treating own family and buddies. At that aspect, it wasn't a commercial enterprise business enterprise choice. I felt better and I desired the people I cherished to sense better too.

Common Signs of SDB in Adults

The maximum common signs of UARS or OSA in adults encompass:

Snoring - Either because of the reality a companion complained or due to the fact they wake themselves up.

Gasping, choking, and save you-breathing episodes - (Usually mentioned with the resource of the use of a companion.)

Falling asleep at the wheel, for quick intervals - This is very volatile and typically a scientific emergency due to the fact vehicle injuries can be lethal.

Nodding off at work - These microsleeps should have an impact on careers, as the sleeper might not appear to be asleep and might conform to assignments while asleep.

Craving salty and candy food and being no longer able to eat healthy food - This is a end end result of the hormone modifications from sleep deprivation. The mind craves fast, best hits to preserve it big huge wide awake.

Lack of energy of thoughts or capacity to make changes - An unrested mind gets stuck in its techniques and it's miles extra difficult to make adjustments, look at new subjects, or increase new behavior.

Weight benefit, and the shortage of capacity to shed pounds despite the fact that dieting and exercise - However, if a person has UARS, they may NOT be overweight however.

High blood strain

Type 2 diabetes or prediabetes

Aching joints and muscle organizations

Waking regularly at night time time

High, slim palate

Overbite

Insomnia, incapability to stay asleep

Anxiety about falling asleep

Treatment-resistant melancholy or tension

Drug or alcohol dependancy. This is frequently self-remedy for sleep problems

Trouble reading more cloth - This symptom regularly shows up even as a person is going lower decrease returned to high school.

Exhaustion, looking commonplace rests in the end of everyday obligations

Brain fog

Large neck duration

Dry mouth in the morning

Waking with a headache

Inability to break out from bed, even after eight hours of "sleep"

Inattention

Irritability

One of the amazing approaches to reveal show display screen an man or woman affected character for SDB, except questionnaires, is to surely spend a few moments speakme to them approximately their lives. Ask for information. How often do they experience exhausted? What duties exhaust them? What did they use a good way to do, that they'll be capable of't anymore? Fleshing out those little information gives a clearer image of the problem, and gives you a manner to offer an explanation for the concrete advantages of getting their sleep troubles dealt with.

www.ingramcontent.com/pod-product-compliance
Lightning Source LLC
Chambersburg PA
CBHW051728020426
42333CB00014B/1206